T0226705

Atopic Dermatitis

Editors

JONATHAN I. SILVERBERG
NANETTE B. SILVERBERG

DERMATOLOGIC CLINICS

www.derm.theclinics.com

Consulting Editor
BRUCE H. THIERS

July 2017 • Volume 35 • Number 3

ELSEVIER

1600 John F. Kennedy Boulevard • Suite 1800 • Philadelphia, Pennsylvania, 19103-2899

http://www.theclinics.com

DERMATOLOGIC CLINICS Volume 35, Number 3
July 2017 ISSN 0733-8635, ISBN-13: 978-0-323-53130-6

Editor: Jessica McCool
Developmental Editor: Alison Swety

© 2017 Elsevier Inc. All rights reserved.

This periodical and the individual contributions contained in it are protected under copyright by Elsevier, and the following terms and conditions apply to their use:

Photocopying
Single photocopies of single articles may be made for personal use as allowed by national copyright laws. Permission of the Publisher and payment of a fee is required for all other photocopying, including multiple or systematic copying, copying for advertising or promotional purposes, resale, and all forms of document delivery. Special rates are available for educational institutions that wish to make photocopies for non-profit educational classroom use. For information on how to seek permission visit www.elsevier.com/permissions or call: (+44) 1865 843830 (UK)/(+1) 215 239 3804 (USA).

Derivative Works
Subscribers may reproduce tables of contents or prepare lists of articles including abstracts for internal circulation within their institutions. Permission of the Publisher is required for resale or distribution outside the institution. Permission of the Publisher is required for all other derivative works, including compilations and translations (please consult www.elsevier. com/permissions).

Electronic Storage or Usage
Permission of the Publisher is required to store or use electronically any material contained in this periodical, including any article or part of an article (please consult www.elsevier.com/permissions). Except as outlined above, no part of this publication may be reproduced, stored in a retrieval system or transmitted in any form or by any means, electronic, mechanical, photocopying, recording or otherwise, without prior written permission of the Publisher.

Notice
No responsibility is assumed by the Publisher for any injury and/or damage to persons or property as a matter of products liability, negligence or otherwise, or from any use or operation of any methods, products, instructions or ideas contained in the material herein. Because of rapid advances in the medical sciences, in particular, independent verification of diagnoses and drug dosages should be made.

Although all advertising material is expected to conform to ethical (medical) standards, inclusion in this publication does not constitute a guarantee or endorsement of the quality or value of such product or of the claims made of it by its manufacturer.

Dermatologic Clinics (ISSN 0733-8635) is published quarterly by Elsevier Inc., 360 Park Avenue South, New York, NY 10010-1710. Months of publication are January, April, July, and October. Business and editorial offices: 1600 John F. Kennedy Blvd., Suite 1800, Philadelphia, PA 19103-2899. Customer service office: 11830 Westline Drive, St. Louis, MO 63146. Periodicals postage paid at New York, NY, and additional mailing offices. Subscription prices are USD 377.00 per year for US individuals, USD 655.00 per year for US institutions, USD 434.00 per year for Canadian individuals, USD 799.00 per year for Canadian institutions, USD 505.00 per year for international individuals, USD 799.00 per year for international institutions, USD 100.00 per year for US students/residents, and USD 240.00 per year for Canadian and international students/residents. International air speed delivery is included in all *Clinics* subscription prices. All prices are subject to change without notice. **POSTMASTER:** Send address changes to *Dermatologic Clinics*, Elsevier Health Sciences Division, Subscription Customer Service, 3251 Riverport Lane, Maryland Heights, MO 63043. **Customer Service: 1-800-654-2452 (U.S. and Canada); 314-447-8871 (outside U.S. and Canada). Fax: 314-447-8029. E-mail: journalscustomerservice-usa@elsevier.com (for print support); journalsonlinesupport-usa@elsevier.com (for online support).**

Reprints. For copies of 100 or more, of articles in this publication, please contact the Commercial Reprints Department, Elsevier Inc., 360 Park Avenue South, New York, New York 10010-1710. Tel.: 212-633-3874; Fax: 212-633-3820; Email: reprints@elsevier.com.

The *Dermatologic Clinics* is covered in *MEDLINE/PubMed (Index Medicus)*, *Current Contents/Clinical Medicine*, *Excerpta Medica*, *Chemical Abstracts,* and *ISI/BIOMED.*

Contributors

CONSULTING EDITOR

BRUCE H. THIERS, MD
Professor and Chairman, Department of
Dermatology and Dermatologic Surgery,
Medical University of South Carolina,
Charleston, South Carolina

EDITORS

JONATHAN I. SILVERBERG, MD, PhD, MPH
Director, Northwestern Medicine
Multidisciplinary Eczema Center, Director,
Contact Dermatitis Clinic, Northwestern
Memorial Hospital, Assistant Professor,
Departments of Dermatology, Preventive
Medicine, and Medical Social Sciences,
Northwestern University Feinberg School of
Medicine, Chicago, Illinois

NANETTE B. SILVERBERG, MD
Chief, Pediatric Dermatology, Mount Sinai
Health Systems, Professor, Departments of
Dermatology and Pediatrics, Icahn School of
Medicine at Mount Sinai, Department of
Dermatology, Mt Sinai St Luke's-Roosevelt
Hospital Center, New York, New York

AUTHORS

KATRINA ABUABARA, MD, MA, MSCE
Assistant Professor, Department of
Dermatology, University of California San
Francisco, San Francisco, California

LISA A. BECK, MD
Dean's Professor of Medicine and
Dermatology, Department of Dermatology,
University of Rochester Medical Center,
Rochester, New York

THOMAS BIEBER, MD, PhD, MDRA
Department of Dermatology and Allergy,
Christine Kühne-Center for Allergy Research
and Education, University Medical Center,
Bonn, Germany

TALI CZARNOWICKI, MD, MSc
Assistant Clinical Professor, Department
of Dermatology, Icahn School of Medicine
at Mount Sinai, Instructor in Clinical
Investigation, Laboratory of Investigative
Dermatology, The Rockefeller University,
New York, New York

AARON M. DRUCKER, MD
Assistant Professor, Department of
Dermatology, Warren Alpert Medical School,
Brown University, Providence, Rhode Island

CAROLA DURÁN-McKINSTER, MD
Department of Pediatric Dermatology,
National Institute of Pediatrics, Mexico City,
Mexico

SARINA B. ELMARIAH, MD, PhD
Assistant Dermatologist, Massachusetts
General Hospital, Instructor, Harvard Medical
School, Boston, Massachusetts

ANNE-SOFIE HALLING-OVERGAARD, MS
Department of Dermatology and Allergy,
Herlev and Gentofte Hospital, University of
Copenhagen, Hellerup, Denmark

JON M. HANIFIN, MD
Professor, Department of Dermatology,
Oregon Health & Science University, Portland,
Oregon

KERRY D. HEITMILLER, BA
University of Maryland School of Medicine,
Baltimore, Maryland

ROBERT KANTOR, MD
Research Fellow, Department of Dermatology,
Northwestern University Feinberg School of
Medicine, Chicago, Illinois

SINÉAD M. LANGAN, FRCP, MSc, PhD
Welcome Senior Clinical Fellow and Associate
Professor, Faculty of Epidemiology and
Population Health, London School of Hygiene
and Tropical Medicine, London, United
Kingdom

KUNAL MALIK, BA
Department of Dermatology, Icahn School of
Medicine at Mount Sinai, Laboratory of
Investigative Dermatology, The Rockefeller
University, New York, New York; SUNY
Downstate College of Medicine, Brooklyn,
New York

DAVID J. MARGOLIS, MD, PhD
Professor, Departments of Dermatology and of
Biostatistics and Epidemiology, University of
Pennsylvania Perelman School of Medicine,
Philadelphia, Pennsylvania

ADELINE MEI-YEN YONG, MRCP (UK)
Resident, Department of Dermatology,
National University Health System, Singapore

JAMES C. PREZZANO, MD
Clinical Research Fellow, Department of
Dermatology, University of Rochester Medical
Center, Rochester, New York

CATHRYN SIBBALD, MD
Division of Dermatology, University of Toronto,
Division of Dermatology, Sunnybrook Health
Sciences Centre, Toronto, Ontario, Canada

JONATHAN I. SILVERBERG, MD, PhD, MPH
Director, Northwestern Medicine
Multidisciplinary Eczema Center, Director,
Contact Dermatitis Clinic, Northwestern
Memorial Hospital, Assistant Professor,
Departments of Dermatology, Preventive
Medicine, and Medical Social Sciences,
Northwestern University Feinberg School of
Medicine, Chicago, Illinois

NANETTE B. SILVERBERG, MD
Chief, Pediatric Dermatology, Mount Sinai
Health Systems, Professor, Departments of
Dermatology and Pediatrics, Icahn School of
Medicine at Mount Sinai, Department of
Dermatology, Mt Sinai St Luke's-Roosevelt
Hospital Center, New York, New York

YONG-KWANG TAY, FRCP (Lond)
Senior Consultant, Department of
Dermatology, Changi General Hospital,
Singapore, Singapore

JACOB P. THYSSEN, MD, PhD, DmSci
Department of Dermatology and Allergy,
Herlev and Gentofte Hospital, National Allergy
Research Centre, Herlev and Gentofte
Hospital, University of Copenhagen, Hellerup,
Denmark

CLAUS ZACHARIAE, MD, DmSci
Department of Dermatology and Allergy,
Herlev and Gentofte Hospital, University of
Copenhagen, Hellerup, Denmark

Contents

Although atopic dermatitis (AD) is the most common skin disorder, there remains an ongoing debate on this denomination, its definition and the binary view based on immunoglobulin E measurement. The wide spectrum of the clinical phenotype of AD reflects the complex genetic and pathophysiologic mechanisms underlying the disease. The diagnostic criteria have to be reconsidered and adapted to different ethnic populations. There is an urgent need for biomarker discovery further supporting the clinical diagnostic criteria as well as the precision medicine approach on a global level.

Atopic dermatitis (AD) is a chronic inflammatory skin disorder with significant morbidity and quality-of-life impairment. The epidemiology of AD is complex and challenging to study. The 1-year US prevalence of AD was 12.98% in children in 2007–2008 and 7.2%–10.2% in adults in 2010–2012. There is considerable statewide and countrywide variation of AD prevalence and severity. The prevalence of childhood AD dramatically increased over the past few decades but may be leveling off in developed nations. AD is associated with increased direct and indirect costs to payers and patients, thereby contributing toward a considerable public health burden.

Atopic dermatitis (AD) is a chronic, relapsing condition, meaning that the intensity of symptoms usually fluctuates over time. Changes in skin physiology may be evident from birth, suggesting that AD may be a lifelong condition marked by intermittent symptoms/disease activity. Methodological considerations for studying the long-term course of AD are reviewed in detail. Improved measurement of the frequency and duration of active disease periods can help to elucidate more about the clinical course AD and the role of treatment in long-term outcomes.

Atopic dermatitis therapy can be a challenge in many cases. Persistence into adulthood often reflects the more severe cases and such patients have the added problems of hand eczema and thick nummular lesions that resist topical medications. Within this group are patients labeled as having adult-onset atopic dermatitis, a designation that is hard to define and probably represents those whose childhood eczema was simply forgotten. Management is difficult for most adult cases and should not be diverted by questionable labels.

Atopic dermatitis is associated with significant patient burden, with impacts from symptoms and visible physical manifestations of the disease. Consequences include detrimental effects on quality of life (QoL), sleep, self-esteem, interpersonal relationships, participation in leisure and sports, and attendance or performance at school or work. Patients also spend a significant amount of time on treatments and care. Worsening severity of disease appears to be associated with a higher risk of impaired QoL, and pharmacologic and educational interventions that improve disease severity appear to, for the most part, simultaneously improve QoL.

Atopic dermatitis (AD) is increasingly recognized as a complex, inflammatory skin disease involving interplay of multiple elements. This article notes key advances in understanding of immune dysregulation, skin barrier dysfunction, environmental, genetic, and microbial influences orchestrating disease pathogenesis, and the relevance of therapeutic interventions in each area. Accumulating evidence and the discovery of new T-cell subsets has matured AD as a multiple-cytokine-axes–driven disorder, evolved from the widely held belief of it being a biphasic Th1/Th2 disease. These new insights have led to active trials testing multiple, targeted therapeutics with better efficacy and safety-profiles.

Moderate to severe atopic dermatitis (AD) can be debilitating and often requires use of systemic immunosuppressant therapy to achieve adequate disease control. There are currently no US Food and Drug Administration–approved systemic agents for the long-term treatment of AD. Recent insight has identified the T helper 2 cytokines, interleukins 4 and 13, as playing a major role in the pathogenesis of AD. There are multiple novel biologic agents in development that target interleukins 4 and/or 13 for the treatment of moderate to severe AD. The age of targeted biologics for AD has arrived.

Many patients with mild to moderate atopic dermatitis (AD) are managed by identifying and avoiding allergens and irritants, ensuring skin moisturization, and graded use of topical corticosteroids and/or calcineurin inhibitors. There is little consensus on the next step. Most systemic therapies are "off label" in the United States and include phototherapy, cyclosporine, mycophenolic acid precursors, azathioprine, and methotrexate. The decision to use these therapies should be based on efficacy and safety readouts from well designed, long-term trials. This article reviews the long-term randomized, controlled trials examining safety and/or efficacy of interventions recommended for patients with mild to severe AD.

Atopic dermatitis is the leading cause of pediatric dermatology visits in developed nations. Recurrent, itchy rashes in typical locations and a family/personal history of atopy helps to identify children with disease. Most cases (85%) are diagnosed by age 5 years. Some comorbidities are age-based and may affect disease course. Topical corticosteroids are the mainstay of therapy; corticosteroidphobia and side effects complicate use. Topical calcineurin inhibitors are alternatives to corticosteroids, especially in sensitive locations. Systemic therapies include antihistamines, immune suppressive agents, and phototherapy, with specific pediatric modifications. This article reviews the nuances and caveats of pediatric atopic dermatitis diagnosis and management.

DERMATOLOGIC CLINICS

ISSUE OF RELATED INTEREST

Immunology & Allergy Clinics, February 2017 (Volume 37, Issue 1)
Allergic Skin Diseases
Peck Y. Ong and Peter Schmid-Grendelmeier, *Editors*
Available at: http://www.immunology.theclinics.com

THE CLINICS ARE AVAILABLE ONLINE!
Access your subscription at:
www.theclinics.com

Preface
Atopic Dermatitis:
A Heterogeneous Disorder

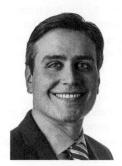

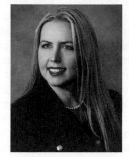

Jonathan I. Silverberg, MD, PhD, MPH   Nanette B. Silverberg, MD

Editors

Atopic dermatitis (AD) is a fascinating disorder. If one had to summarize AD in one word, perhaps the best descriptor would be "heterogeneity." That is, all aspects of the disease, including its name, epidemiology, clinical course, and treatment approaches, have a considerable amount of heterogeneity. Such heterogeneity begs the question, is AD one disease or a spectrum of diseases with a shared phenotype? Much of the scientific and clinical literature about AD has been relegated to childhood disease, with limited data available even in that subgroup. As it turns out, AD may be far more common in adults than previously recognized, whether through persistence or adult onset. Little is known about AD in adults. Is it the same disease as pediatric AD or not?

AD can be hard to define and diagnose (particularly in adults) given its many clinical presentations. Thomas Bieber masterfully reviews the heterogeneous definitions used for AD, how valid they are, and the impact of their use in different settings. Moreover, Professor Bieber provides important perspective on the future of molecular diagnostics and a more refined definition of AD. This outlook will in the future clarify the true nature of disease and allow us to project to patients a more accurate view of their clinical future.

AD is one of the most burdensome of all skin disorders globally, owing to its high prevalence and patient burden. Jonathan Silverberg reviews the public health burden and epidemiology of pediatric and adult AD. The burden of AD now rivals the impact of many chronic illnesses and identifies AD as a serious and even a systemic condition.

AD is a chronic disorder that can have a heterogeneous clinical course. For some, the disease is more episodic or seasonal, while others can have a more chronic persistent course. Children with AD may have persistent disease well into adulthood. Katrina Abuabara and colleagues review the long-term course of AD, how to define different concepts pertaining to a longitudinal course of AD, and their relevance in different settings. Many studies have shown high rates of self-reported adult-onset disease. However, the matter of adult-onset AD remains quite controversial. Jon Hanifin discusses whether adult-onset AD is fact or fancy. This is a very clinically relevant question because the differential diagnosis of adult-onset AD is quite broad and difficult to rule out.

There are important AD patient subsets that require special consideration with respect to both assessment and management. AD is likely not one illness, but a constellation of linked cutaneous manifestations that appear throughout a lifetime. Professors Nanette Silverberg and Carola Durán-McKinster review important physical manifestations, comorbidities, and treatment considerations in pediatric AD. Yong-Kwang Tay and Adeline Mei-Yen Yong review important racial and ethnic differences of AD epidemiology, phenotype, distribution, severity, genetics, and even treatment. Recognition of AD as clinically variable by age, race, and ethnicity highlights the variable roles that genetics and environment play on the emergence of clinical features and therapeutic outcomes.

The profound symptom-burden and heterogeneous manifestations of AD negatively impact

Dermatol Clin 35 (2017) ix–x
http://dx.doi.org/10.1016/j.det.2017.04.001
0733-8635/17/© 2017 Published by Elsevier Inc.

upon quality of life in a variety of ways. Aaron Drucker and Cathryn Sibbald review the impact of the profound symptom burden and stigma of AD on quality of life. The quality of life impairment appears to be directly related to AD severity in most cases and in turn warrants improved prevention strategies and better long-term disease control, the latter being the holy grail of AD care.

James Prezzano and Lisa Beck comprehensively review long-term treatment strategies for chronic AD, including skin care recommendations, proactive topical therapy, long-term safety and efficacy of topical corticosteroids and calcinuerin inhibitors, phototherapy, and systemic immunosuppressants.

Pruritus or itch is the hallmark symptom of AD and can be very challenging to treat, often failing to clear with sedating antihistamines, which may be associated with undesirable side effects. Sarina Elmariah reviews the impact of current standard of care topical and/or systemic therapies on pruritus. Furthermore, she reviews a variety of adjunctive anti-itch strategies, including topical agents, antiepileptics, antidepressants, neurokinin-1 receptor antagonists, opioid modulators, and alternative therapies.

Jacob Thyssen and colleagues review the diagnostic and therapeutic considerations for yet another important patient subset, atopic hand eczema. Hand eczema can develop secondary to lower irritant threshold or superimposed allergic contact dermatitis in persons with AD. This is a very clinically relevant and important subset because failure to adequately avoid exogenous triggers may result in treatment-refractory hand eczema.

The last decade has witnessed major strides in our understanding of the pathogenesis of AD. Tali Czarnowicki and colleagues do a wonderful job reviewing the pathways implicated in the pathophysiology, barrier disruption, and immune dysregulation of AD. One of the most promising new developments in our understanding of AD is the recognition that AD is an immune-mediated disorder largely driven by T-helper 2 cytokines,

interleukin-4, and/or interleukin-13. Jonathan Silverberg and Robert Kantor review the role of interleukin-4 and/or interleukin-13 in the pathogenesis of AD. These insights have directly translated into the development of novel biologic agents targeting these cytokine pathways. The first such biologic agent to be approved by the US Food and Drug Administration for AD was dupilumab, with multiple other biologic, systemic, and topical agents in the pipeline for AD.

AD has just begun to command the respect it deserves as a chronic disease with negative life impact and comorbidities. The future holds new definitions, better recognition of disease manifestations, superior surveillance for comorbidities, and an impressive improvement in therapeutic interventions. This is truly an exciting time for patients with AD, the people who suffer with them, and clinicians who treat AD.

Jonathan I. Silverberg, MD, PhD, MPH
Northwestern Medicine
Multidisciplinary Eczema Center
Contact Dermatitis Clinic
Northwestern Memorial Hospital
Departments of Dermatology, Preventive
Medicine, and Medical Social Sciences
Northwestern University
Feinberg School of Medicine
676 North Saint Clair Street
Suite 1600
Chicago, IL 60611, USA

Nanette B. Silverberg, MD
Pediatric Dermatology
Mount Sinai Health Systems
Departments of Dermatology and Pediatrics
Icahn School of Medicine at Mount Sinai
425 West 59th Street
Suite 8B
New York, NY 10019, USA

E-mail addresses:
jonathanisilverberg@gmail.com (J.I. Silverberg)
nsilverb@chpnet.org (N.B. Silverberg)

How to Define Atopic Dermatitis?

Thomas Bieber, MD, PhD, MDRA

KEYWORDS

• Atopic dermatitis • Eczema • Definition • Immunoglobuline E • Precision medicine

KEY POINTS

• Atopic dermatitis (AD) display a wide clinical phenotype, varying according to ethnic populations.
• The value of total immunoglobulin E as a single biomarker for atopy and/or the diagnosis of AD is questionable.
• We need a refinement of the diagnostic criteria for AD according to ethnic populations.
• Research should focus on the discovery and validation of biomarkers for a precision medicine approach improving the definition and clinical diagnosis of AD.
• Future biomarkers will allow a better stratification of AD for personalized prevention and therapeutic approaches.

INTRODUCTION

Atopic dermatitis (AD) is a paradigmatic disease that has always challenged the scientific community with regard to its origin and the wide spectrum of the clinical phenotype. The multiple denominations for this disease over the last century underline this lack of consensus with regard overall to the understanding of the origin of the disease.[1–4] The term AD was coined by Wise and Sulzberger in 1933[5] and has merely adopted over the time. In the last 2 decades or so, there have been a number of attempts to redefine the disease according to more modern insights based on epidemiologic studies, genetic findings as well as immunologic pathomechanisms underlying the disease.

Without going much into the discussion of whether or not the term AD is the most suitable one for this condition, one should notice that it has been always a tradition in medicine and particularly in dermatology that designations of the diseases usually are based on a composite name typically relying to a symptom on one hand and an adjective for the context of that symptom on the other. Typical examples for this kind of denomination are *mycosis fungoides, lichen planus, psoriasis vulgaris, lupus erythematodes* or in our particular case, *atopic dermatitis*. The scientific community nowadays acknowledges the complexity of the clinical phenotype and of the pathophysiologic background of AD. The phenotype may rather correspond with a common set of symptoms that the skin has found in his own language to express the various underlying mechanisms that we just start to understand. The term "skin disease" has recently been proposed for this particular situation.[6]

IS IT *ECZEMA* OR *DERMATITIS*?

Interestingly, although physicians mean the same syndromic situation called herein AD, depending on the countries the preferred name can be different and this phenomenon certainly has a significant impact for many different aspects of practical relevance.[1,4] For example, the term *eczema* is more commonly used in the UK and in countries of the Commonwealth, whereas *atopic eczema* and *atopic dermatitis* are rather used and mixed up in other countries. A particular situation is observed

Disclosure Statement: The author has no relevant conflict of interest for this article.
Department of Dermatology and Allergy, Christine Kühne-Center for Allergy Research and Education, University Medical Center, Sigmund-Freud-Street 25, Bonn 53127, Germany
E-mail address: Thomas.Bieber@ukb.uni-bonn.de

derm.theclinics.com

in China, where *eczema* and *atopic dermatitis* are considered as 2 different diseases (see below). Sticking to the original meaning of the word *eczema*, coming from the Greek word εκσειν (eksein), which means "boiling," this denomination, particularly without the adjective *atopic*, seems the less suitable because it strongly suggests a disease in an acute situation with vesicles as a major clinical sign. Based on that and with regard to the classical clinical symptoms of this condition, the word *eczema* would seem the less appropriate for this disease, in particular when the adjective *atopic* is not combined. Therefore, a new discussion has been started on an global level with the aim to harmonize at least the denomination of the condition because this is expected to have significant relevance for a more global approach in terms of research, education, prevention, and drug development.[4]

HOW TO DEFINE *ATOPY*?

Beside the wording *eczema* or *dermatitis*, the definition of *atopy* is probably much more challenging. When facing the particular situation of a special familiar hyperresponsiveness against allergens, Coca and Cooke[7] asked the philologist Edward Perry to find a suitable term. Finally, they agree to the artificial term atopy which is derived from the Greek word ατοποσ (atopos) and means "not in the right place, not in the precise place, unusual, strange." Since then, this nonmedical term survived overtime and has been accepted to describe this particular kind of syndrome including an involvement of different target organs, such as the skin, lung, nose, and/or eyes, while the immune system seems to mount a specific immunity with immunoglobulin E (IgE). However, although there is a consensus about what the scientific community overall means by *atopy*, there remains a never-ending discussion on how to best define this in a consensual definition. For instance, the probably best definition of atopy remains the following: "atopy is a personal and/or family tendency to become sensitized and produce IgE antibodies in response to ordinary exposures to allergens, usually proteins. As a consequence, these individuals can develop typical symptoms of asthma, rhino-conjunctivitis and eczema/dermatitis."[8] The dilemma of this definition is that most of the scientists would stick to the proof on an IgE-mediated sensitization in a distinct individual to apply the term atopy. However, in the given definition, it seems obvious that the production of IgE is a consequence of this predisposition, and not the origin. This subtle distinction is of particular significance when it comes to consider the very

early phase of AD, where a given individual starts to have typical clinical symptoms of the disease but the sensitization against environmental allergens cannot yet be detected because it is expected to appear during the course of the disease.[9] Therefore, the very early phase of AD in infancy (phase 1) is related to an atopic predisposition even if increased total IgE and/or specific IgE cannot yet be demonstrated, at least with the available panel of allergens and technologies.

WHAT ABOUT *INTRINSIC* VERSUS *EXTRINSIC* ATOPIC DERMATITIS?

Among the patients suffering from typical clinical symptoms compatible with the diagnosis of AD, there seems to be a subgroup in which the patients lack increased total IgE or specific IgE to common allergens. Interestingly, the same phenomenon as described for the disease itself with multiple different denominations, is reproduced for this particular subgroup for which different terms have been coined such as intrinsic AD,[10] *atopy form* dermatitis,[11,12] or *non–IgE-associated* dermatitis or *nonatopic eczema*.[8] As mentioned, normal IgE and/or the lack of detectable specific IgE can be encountered mainly in 2 situations: (i) in infancy or early childhood when the clinical dermatologic symptoms are present, but the sensitization process has not yet led to the generation of increased IgE synthesis.[13,14] Interestingly, many studies have highlighted the fact that the situation is more frequent in female individuals than in males.[15,16] Similarly, (ii) in the so-called late onset of the disease, this particular form affects mainly females with a rather mild form of the disease, emerging in the absence of increased total IgE or seemingly detectable specific IgE.[16,17] There is currently no convincing explanation for the fact that IgE sensitization occurs earlier and in a more pronounced way in males than in females.

However, the existence of a non–IgE-associated form of AD can be strongly questioned.[18] Indeed, the cutoff for the so called 'normal IgE' has been fixed at around 100 kU/L.[19] In contrast, the exploration of specific IgE is limited to a distinct more or less large panel of common allergens. Thus, we will always face the typical issue of the limitation of the value of IgE as a reliable biomarker to appreciate the atopic status of a patient and his very individual and personalized sensitization profile. In fact, most physicians have frequently faced the situation of patients with normal total IgE (<100 kU/L) but clear-cut oligosensitization to some relevant allergens such as house dust mite or pollens with significant proportion of specific IgE within this normal total IgE amount. This kind of oligosensitization is most probably of much more clinical relevance for a given individual compared with other patients with very high IgE level (>1000 kU/L) and a wide spectrum of the so-called specific IgE as measured by radioallergosorbent test. Therefore, not only the cutoff of total IgE may seriously be questioned, but also the panel of allergens used in the detection of the individual sensitization profile.

Moreover, we always use the term 'specific IgE' in our scientific discourse. This term is used usually because we have a tremendous gap between the sum of the so-called specific IgE amount and the total IgE level in many patients with high overall IgE levels. Clearly, in the 1970s, when the detection of specific IgE and the availability of purified allergen for this detection was rather limited, the panel of possible allergens and the detection of specific IgE was rather limited.[20] With time and new technologies, including the availability of recombinant allergens,[21] the panel of available allergens for exploring the sensitization profile of a given individual has increased dramatically. Thus, owing to technical progress in in vitro diagnostics, the spectrum of possible specific IgE is increasing whereas the spectrum of the so-called non-IgE within the total IgE amount is gradually decreasing. In this regard, a key statement should be considered: There is no "nonspecific IgE"; there is only IgE from which we do not yet know the specificity!

From these considerations, the binary view of AD and the existence of a non-IgE-associated (intrinsic, atopiform, etc) can be seriously questioned.[22] Indeed, a more thorough exploration of the specific IgE particularly for microbial agents or self-proteins[23] in individuals with normal total IgE (according to the current cut-off point) would probably allow to detect some level of sensitization in each individual affected by AD.[24]

Another important aspect that supports this exposed concept is the fact that there is a well-established correlation between the severity of the disease and at least the amount of total IgE.[25] More recently, some transcriptomic analyses of intrinsic forms of AD have shown partly conflicting results.[26–28] The differences more rely on the expression of other cytokines like Th-22 and Th-17, which may potentially counterbalance the Th-2 dominance in terms of IgE synthesis and, therefore, limit at least to some point the ongoing sensitization mechanisms in these individuals. Similarly, differences in FLG mutations do not seem to fully explain the phenomenon.[27] Our clinical experience also shows that although there may be some patients who show an increase in severity by the time in the early phase of the disease, particularly in childhood, in many instances the degree of severity of a given patient is a rather stable phenomenon, which seems to be an important factor in driving the sensitization phenomenon. The key question of the future will be to identify the mechanisms responsible for driving the severity and to find suitable and related biomarkers with a prognostic or predictive value for these individuals.

IMPACT OF THE DEFINITION ON THE DIAGNOSTIC CRITERIA FOR ATOPIC DERMATITIS

Since the first diagnostic criteria from Hanifin and Rajka in the early 1980s,[29] a number of other diagnostic criteria more or less based on the latter, have been proposed and listed on **Table 1**. A comparative view of the "must have" in the 3 most used criteria, that is, the Hanifin and Rajka, the UK working party and the criteria from the American Academy of Dermatology (**Table 2**) shows the different perceptions of the individual diagnostic items with regard to the qualitative

Table 1
Diagnostic criteria for atopy and atopic dermatitis

Criteria	Year	References
Wise and Sulzberger	1933	5
Hanifin and Rajka	1980	29
Kang and Tian Diagnostic criteria	1987	42
UK Working Party	1994	33
Lillehammer criteria	1996	31
Japanese Dermatological Association Guidelines	1995	32
International Study of Asthma and Allergy in Childhood	1995	43
Diepgen criteria	1996	31
Millennium criteria	1998	44
Indian guidelines	2001	36
Thai criteria in children	2004	45
Danish Allergy Research Centre	2005	46
Thai criteria in adults	2007	35
American Academy of Dermatology Guidelines	2014	34
Chinese criteria (adolescents/adults)	2016	37
Korean Atopic Dermatitis Research Group Criteria	2016	47

Table 2
Comparison of the "must have" (qualitative major criteria) items in the 3 common diagnostic criteria

Aspects Considered	Hanifin & Rajka,[29] 1980	UK Working Party,[33] 1994	American Academy of Dermatology,[34] 2014
Morphology and distribution	• Flexural lichenification in adults • Facial and extensor involvement in infants and children	• History of involvement of the skin creases (elbows, knees, ankles, neck) • Visible flexural eczema	Eczema Typical morphology Age-specific patterns
Chronicity	Chronic or chronically relapsing dermatitis		Chronic or relapsing history
History	Personal or family history of atopy (asthma, allergic rhinitis, atopic dermatitis)	• Personal history of asthma or hay fever or • History of atopic disease in a first-degree relative	
Pruritus		Itchy skin condition	Pruritus
Dry skin		History of dry skin in the last year	
Onset		Under the age of 2	

major criteria used. The value of qualitative versus quantitative AD criteria is of great importance and has been excellently discussed in details elsewhere.[30] A first short survey performed in 2016 across Europe, the United States, and Asian countries including Japan, Korea, Thailand, and China has shown that the use of diagnostic criteria is very much dependent on the context in which the diagnosis of AD must be ascertained (Bieber, personal communication, 2016). Although in most clinical trials the criteria of Hanifin and Rajka are still considered as the gold standard, the situation is by far different when it comes to the first choice of diagnostic criteria in a routine work. Interestingly, the Diepgen criteria[31] are only used in Europe. The Japanese Dermatological Association criteria[32] are mainly used in Japan, but also to some extend in China. The UK Working Party[33] criteria are mainly used in Europe and in China but not in the United States. In the United States, the criteria of the American Academy of Dermatology[34] are the preferred ones. As expected, some national criteria, such as in Thailand[35] and India,[36] are primarily used in these countries.

What can we learn from this short survey? The fact that so many national societies are by the time generating their own diagnostic criteria may reflect 2 main aspects: (i) Hanifin and Rajka criteria are complex, time consuming and therefore not the first choice for the routine work. Therefore, other criteria representing a simplified form of the Hanifin and Rajka criteria, such as the UK Working Party criteria seems more preferable for this purpose. In contrast, (ii) one should also consider

that the criteria proposed in the Hanifin and Rajka or UK Working Party may well fit for the Caucasian population but may not be applicable for the clinical phenotype of AD in all ethnic populations. This seems particularly true for the situation in some Asian countries like Japan and China.

Moreover, among all of these world regions, the situation in China is of particular interest. For different reasons, partly of cultural and historical origin, such as the traditional Chinese medicine, the Chinese physicians have divided the clinical phenotype of AD in 2 distinct entities: (i) eczema and (ii) AD. For a given patient affected by the disease, a stringent application of the Hanifin and Rajka criteria will lead to the classification into either eczema when the requested criteria are not fulfilled (eg, family history is missing), or AD when the criteria are fulfilled. This particular dichotic view of the clinical phenotype may have led to a substantial underestimation of the incidence of this disease in this particular country in the past. A recent analysis of the different criteria applied to a population of adult and adolescent patients with AD has shown that indeed the sensitivity of the classical Hanifin and Rajka criteria as well as the UK Working Party criteria is much less compared with the newly defined criteria for the Chinese population.[37]

Several conclusions can be drawn with regard to the diagnostic criteria currently in use worldwide. As has been suggested by Asian dermatologists, we may have to revise the classical criteria according to the different ethnic populations taking into consideration some particularities that may have distinct genetic origins.[37,38] Beside the particular situation in China and Korea, similar adaptations of the criteria may be needed in other Asian countries as well as in the African and American population or possibly in South America. With regard to the globalization of science and translational medicine up to drug development, a dialogue between the different dermatologic communities with regard to the diagnostic criteria for AD to be used in the future in the context of epidemiologic studies, global research, programs and pharmaceutical developments is urgently needed.

WHAT COULD BE THE CONTRIBUTION OF PRECISION MEDICINE IN A REFINED DEFINITION AND DIAGNOSIS OF ATOPIC DERMATITIS?

As mentioned, we still have a number of unsolved issues with regard to the application of the diagnostic criteria on a global level as well as for the 2 edges of the lifespan, (i) in the very early phase in infancy before 6 months and, in contrast, (ii) in elderly (in the so-called silver generation). To improve the diagnostic criteria for global studies, we need a refinement of the criteria with some degree of adaptation to the different ethnic populations. To achieve this goal, which represents a substantial challenge for the scientific community, we ideally will need concerted efforts in recruiting large cohorts of patients worldwide, to collect clinical and exposome data, as well as biological material of these individuals and to follow them up to better understand the natural history of the disease and the phenotypic particularities in different ethnic populations. Moreover, the patient registries in combination with the data generated from the biobanks in a systems biology approach will allow the discovery of new diagnostic biomarkers and will allow a reliable phenotype–endophenotype relationship.[39] This material will also be the basement for the future molecular taxonomy of AD, the discovery and validation of biomarkers for screening purposes enabling stratification of the population at risk and targeted prevention approaches.[40] Finally, some of these biomarkers will also have prognostic and predictive value with regard to the evolution of the disease, the occurrence of the atopic march and potentially to the responsiveness to the newly developed drugs targeting the most dominant pathways underlying the different phenotypes.[41]

SUMMARY AND PERSPECTIVES

AD is the most common skin disease encountered in daily practice for dermatologists, pediatricians,

and perhaps for other disciplines as well. It seems ironic that there is no harmonization so far with regard to the name of this condition and that the classical diagnostic criteria may not be applicable worldwide. A harmonized umbrella term 'atopic dermatitis' will be able to include many subforms, which will be defined in the future by biomarker-based stratification. Moreover, we will have to consider the variations of the clinical phenotype according to the ethnic populations and to work on refined criteria for a better understanding of the disease and better prevention and therapeutic approaches on a global level. Although the clinical phenotype of AD represents a wide spectrum, attempts to dissect this disease in different autonomous entities based solely on the use of total or specific IgE may eventually fail. Instead, we have to consider AD not only clinically but also from a pathophysiologic point of view as a wide spectrum of complex mechanisms that are most probably overlapping at the level of the barrier dysfunction and/or the innate and adapted immune system. The genetically driven dominance of distinct parts of this pathophysiologic relevant mechanisms may lead to particularities in the clinical phenotype and ultimately for diagnostic criteria as well as for prevention and therapeutic approaches.

REFERENCES

1. Kantor R, Thyssen JP, Paller AS, et al. Atopic dermatitis, atopic eczema, or eczema? A systematic review, meta-analysis, and recommendation for uniform use of 'atopic dermatitis'. Allergy 2016;71(10):1480–5.
2. Taieb A, Hanifin J, Cooper K, et al. Proceedings of the 4th Georg Rajka International Symposium on Atopic Dermatitis, Arcachon, France, September 15-17, 2005. J Allergy Clin Immunol 2006;117(2):378–90.
3. Wallach D, Taieb A, Tilles G. Histoire de la dermatite atopique. Paris: Masson; 2005. p. 284.
4. Bieber T. Why we need a harmonized name for atopic dermatitis/atopic eczema/eczema! Allergy 2016;71(10):1379–80.
5. Wise F, Sulzberger M. Year Book of Dermatology and Syphilology 1933.
6. Wallach D. The significance of atopic dermatitis. J Dermatol Res 2016;1:1–5.
7. Coca A, Cooke R. On the classification of the phenomenon of hypersensitiveness. J Immunol 1923;8: 163–82.
8. Johansson SG, Bieber T, Dahl R, et al. Revised nomenclature for allergy for global use: report of the nomenclature review committee of the world allergy organization, October 2003. J Allergy Clin Immunol 2004;113(5):832–6.
9. Bieber T. Atopic dermatitis. Ann Dermatol 2010; 22(2):125–37.

10. Schmid-Grendelmeier P, Simon D, Simon HU, et al. Epidemiology, clinical features, and immunology of the "intrinsic" (non-IgE-mediated) type of atopic dermatitis (constitutional dermatitis). Allergy 2001; 56(9):841–9.

11. Bos JD. Atopiform dermatitis. Br J Dermatol 2002; 147(3):426–9.

12. Bos JD, Brenninkmeijer EE, Schram ME, et al. Atopic eczema or atopiform dermatitis. Exp Dermatol 2010; 19(4):325–31.

13. Illi S, von Mutius E, Lau S, et al. The natural course of atopic dermatitis from birth to age 7 years and the association with asthma. J Allergy Clin Immunol 2004;113(5):925–31.

14. Park JH, Choi YL, Namkung JH, et al. Characteristics of extrinsic vs. intrinsic atopic dermatitis in infancy: correlations with laboratory variables. Br J Dermatol 2006;155(4):778–83.

15. Brenninkmeijer EE, Spuls PI, Legierse CM, et al. Clinical differences between atopic and atopiform dermatitis. J Am Acad Dermatol 2008;58(3): 407–14.

16. Zeppa L, Bellini V, Lisi P. Atopic dermatitis in adults. Dermatitis 2011;22(1):40–6.

17. Tokura Y. Extrinsic and intrinsic types of atopic dermatitis. J Dermatol Sci 2010;58(1):1–7.

18. Folster-Holst R, Pape M, Buss YL, et al. Low prevalence of the intrinsic form of atopic dermatitis among adult patients. Allergy 2006;61(5):629–32.

19. Ott H, Stanzel S, Ocklenburg C, et al. Total serum IgE as a parameter to differentiate between intrinsic and extrinsic atopic dermatitis in children. Acta Derm Venereol 2009;89(3):257–61.

20. Church JA, Kleban DG, Bellanti JA. Serum immunoglobulin E concentrations and radioallergosorbent tests in children with atopic dermatitis. Pediatr Res 1976;10(2):97–9.

21. Onell A, Whiteman A, Nordlund B, et al. Allergy testing in children with persistent asthma: comparison of four diagnostic methods. Allergy 2017;72(4): 590–7.

22. Karimkhani C, Silverberg JI, Dellavalle RP. Defining intrinsic vs. extrinsic atopic dermatitis. Dermatol Online J 2015;21(6).

23. Mothes N, Niggemann B, Jenneck C, et al. The cradle of IgE autoreactivity in atopic eczema lies in early infancy. J Allergy Clin Immunol 2005;116(3): 706–9.

24. Novak N, Allam JP, Bieber T. Allergic hyperreactivity to microbial components: a trigger factor of "intrinsic" atopic dermatitis? J Allergy Clin Immunol 2003;112(1):215–6.

25. Berg T, Johansson SG. IgE concentrations in children with atopic diseases. A clinical study. Int Arch Allergy Appl Immunol 1969;36(3):219–32.

26. Suarez-Farinas M, Dhingra N, Gittler J, et al. Intrinsic atopic dermatitis shows similar TH2 and higher TH17 immune activation compared with extrinsic atopic dermatitis. J Allergy Clin Immunol 2013; 132(2):361–70.

27. Martel BC, Litman T, Hald A, et al. Distinct molecular signatures of mild extrinsic and intrinsic atopic dermatitis. Exp Dermatol 2016;25(6):453–9.

28. Kabashima-Kubo R, Nakamura M, Sakabe J, et al. A group of atopic dermatitis without IgE elevation or barrier impairment shows a high Th1 frequency: possible immunological state of the intrinsic type. J Dermatol Sci 2012;67(1):37–43.

29. Hanifin J, Rajka G. Diagnostic features of atopic eczema. Acta Derm Venereol 1980;92:44–7.

30. Andersen RM, Thyssen JP, Maibach HI. Qualitative vs. quantitative atopic dermatitis criteria - in historical and present perspectives. J Eur Acad Dermatol Venereol 2016;30(4):604–18.

31. Diepgen TL, Sauerbrei W, Fartasch M. Development and validation of diagnostic scores for atopic dermatitis incorporating criteria of data quality and practical usefulness. J Clin Epidemiol 1996;49(9): 1031–8.

32. Tagami H. Japanese dermatological association criteria for the diagnosis of atopic dermatitis. J Dermatol 1995;22:966–7.

33. Williams HC, Burney PG, Hay RJ, et al. The U.K. working party's diagnostic criteria for atopic dermatitis. I. Derivation of a minimum set of discriminators for atopic dermatitis. Br J Dermatol 1994;131(3): 383–96.

34. Eichenfield LF, Tom WL, Chamlin SL, et al. Guidelines of care for the management of atopic dermatitis: section 1. Diagnosis and assessment of atopic dermatitis. J Am Acad Dermatol 2014;70(2): 338–51.

35. Wanitphakdeedecha R, Tuchinda P, Sivayathorn A, et al. Validation of the diagnostic criteria for atopic dermatitis in the adult Thai population. Asian Pac J Allergy Immunol 2007;25(2–3):133–8.

36. Sharma L. Diagnostic clinical features of atopic dermatitis. Indian J Dermatol Venereol Leprol 2001; 67(1):25–7.

37. Liu P, Zhao Y, Mu ZL, et al. Clinical features of adult/ adolescent atopic dermatitis and Chinese criteria for atopic dermatitis. Chin Med J (Engl) 2016;129(7): 757–62.

38. Lee HJ, Cho SH, Ha SJ, et al. Minor cutaneous features of atopic dermatitis in South Korea. Int J Dermatol 2000;39(5):337–42.

39. Bieber T, Akdis C, Lauener R, et al. Global allergy forum and 3rd Davos declaration 2015: atopic dermatitis/eczema: challenges and opportunities toward precision medicine. Allergy 2016;71(5): 588–92.

40. Bieber T. Atopic dermatitis 2.0: from the clinical phenotype to the molecular taxonomy and stratified medicine. Allergy 2012;67(12):1475–82.

41. Bieber T, Vieths S, Broich K. New opportunities and challenges in the assessment of drugs for atopic diseases. Allergy 2016;71(12):1662–5.

42. Kang KF, Tian RM. Atopic dermatitis. An evaluation of clinical and laboratory findings. Int J Dermatol 1987;26(1):27–32.

43. Asher MI, Keil U, Anderson HR, et al. International study of asthma and allergies in childhood (ISAAC): rationale and methods. Eur Respir J 1995;8(3): 483–91.

44. Bos JD, Van Leent EJ, Sillevis Smitt JH. The millennium criteria for the diagnosis of atopic dermatitis. Exp Dermatol 1998;7(4):132–8.

45. Wisuthsarewong W, Viravan S. Diagnostic criteria for atopic dermatitis in Thai children. J Med Assoc Thai 2004;87(12):1496–500.

46. Johnke H, Vach W, Norberg LA, et al. A comparison between criteria for diagnosing atopic eczema in infants. Br J Dermatol 2005;153(2):352–8.

47. Lee SC, Committee of Korean Atopic Dermatitis Association for REACH. Various diagnostic criteria for atopic dermatitis (AD): a proposal of reliable estimation of atopic dermatitis in childhood (REACH) criteria, a novel questionnaire-based diagnostic tool for AD. J Dermatol 2016; 43(4):376–84.

Public Health Burden and Epidemiology of Atopic Dermatitis

Jonathan I. Silverberg, MD, PhD, MPH[a,b,c],*

KEYWORDS

- Atopic dermatitis • Eczema • Epidemiology • Cost • Children • Adult • Severity • Prevalence

KEY POINTS

- Atopic dermatitis (AD) poses a significant public health burden owing to its high prevalence, considerable morbidity, increased health care utilization, and cost of care.
- AD may be more common in adults than previously recognized, secondary to both persistence of childhood disease and adult-onset disease.
- The prevalence of childhood atopic dermatitis dramatically increased in the United States and internationally over the past few years.
- Recent studies suggest that atopic dermatitis is more common in adults than previously thought.
- Atopic dermatitis is associated with a considerable public health burden owing to its very high prevalence, considerable patient-burden and increased healthcare utilization.

INTRODUCTION

AD is a chronic inflammatory skin disease affecting both children and adults. AD is associated with a substantial public health burden secondary to high prevalence in many regions and increased health care utilization and costs. The epidemiology of AD has evolved over the past few decades, with emerging trends and novel insights into the burden of disease. Studying the epidemiology of AD is complex. This review addresses recent developments in the epidemiology and public health burden of AD.

CHALLENGES OF STUDYING THE EPIDEMIOLOGY OF ATOPIC DERMATITIS

There are several challenges of studying the epidemiology of AD. First, there are no widely accepted biomarkers or objective diagnostic tests for AD. Moreover, the lack of standardized nomenclature for AD internationally, for example, atopic neurodermatitis, eczema, atopic eczema, and childhood eczema, makes it difficult to develop consistent and valid questionnaires for epidemiology research. In particular, the term, *eczema*, has several different uses, including as the most commonly used lay synonym for AD, as a descriptive morphologic and/or histologic term encompassing multiple etiologies, and as a diagnostic term for AD.[1] Furthermore, there is considerable heterogeneity of AD with respect to the distribution (eg, flexural, extensor, head and neck areas, and generalized), morphology (eg, oozing, scaling, lichenification, prurigo nodules, ill-demarcated, and psoriasiform), intensity and time course (intermittent, chronic persistent disease,

The author has nothing to disclose.
[a] Department of Dermatology, Northwestern University Feinberg School of Medicine, 676 North Street Clair Street, Suite 1600, Chicago, IL 60611, USA; [b] Department of Preventive Medicine, Northwestern University Feinberg School of Medicine, Chicago, IL 60611, USA; [c] Department of Medical Social Sciences, Northwestern University Feinberg School of Medicine, Chicago, IL 60611, USA
* Northwestern Medicine Multidisciplinary Eczema Center, 676 North Street Clair Street, Suite 1600, Chicago, IL 60611.
E-mail address: JonathanISilverberg@gmail.com

Dermatol Clin 35 (2017) 283–289
http://dx.doi.org/10.1016/j.det.2017.02.002
0733-8635/17/© 2017 Elsevier Inc. All rights reserved.

seasonal variation, and episodic flares), and associated comorbidities. As such, numerous approaches have been used to assess the epidemiology of AD, but there is no universally valid approach.

EPIDEMIOLOGY OF CHILDHOOD ATOPIC DERMATITIS
United States

Recent prevalence estimates of childhood AD in the United States range from 6% to 12.98%, depending on the study design and approach used to assess for AD. A household survey of 42,249 children and adults in 1998 found that 10.7% had empirically defined eczema, and 6% had empirically defined AD.[2] This study did not distinguish, however, between AD in children and adults. Household surveys of 102,353 and 91,642 children ages 0 to 17 from the 2003–2004 National Survey of Children's Health (NSCH) and 2007–2008 NSCH found the 1-year prevalence of caregiver-reported health care–diagnosed eczema to be 10.7% and 12.98%, respectively, with significant variation between states and districts (8.7%–18.1%)[3,4] (**Fig. 1**A). The question used to assess AD was subsequently validated and found to have good sensitivity and excellent specificity and positive predictive value.[5] Comparison between 2003–2004 and 2007–2008 suggests that the prevalence of childhood AD is increasing over time. Data from the National Health Interview Survey (NHIS), a US population-based household survey, indicate that the prevalence of childhood AD steadily increased from approximately 8% in 1997 to more than 12% in 2010 and 2011 but may have plateaued in 2012 and 2013 (**Fig. 2**).

Several sociodemographic groups seem at higher risk for childhood AD in the United States. Several studies found higher prevalence of AD in African Americans/blacks, even after controlling for several potential confounding factors, such as household income, health insurance coverage, and parental education level.[4,6] Multiple US population-based studies found no association between gender and AD.[3,7] Children from the NSCH study also had a higher prevalence of caregiver-reported AD with increased household incomes, higher family education levels, smaller family sizes, and urban and metropolitan living.[3]

International

Many studies have been performed to determine the prevalence of childhood AD in other countries around the world. It is often difficult, however, to compare the results of such studies owing to disparate study designs, sampling methodologies, and definitions of AD. Some of the best estimates of AD prevalence internationally were generated from the International Study of Asthma and Allergies in Childhood (ISAAC). This international epidemiologic research collaboration provided a global map of AD, allowing for comparison of prevalence estimates between different countries by consistently using a modified version of the United Kingdom Working Party criteria to define AD.[8] Odhiambo and colleagues[8] analyzed data from 385,853 participants ages 6 to 7 and 663,256 participants ages 13 to 14 in the ISAAC Phase 3 study. They found a wide variation in prevalence values worldwide, from 0.9% in India to 22.5% in Ecuador at ages 6 years to 7 years and from 0.2% in China to 24.6% in Colombia at ages 13 years to 14 years. Comparison of prevalence estimates between Phases 1 and 3 of the ISAAC study suggest increasing prevalence of AD among 6 year olds to 7 year olds in both developing and developed nations and increasing prevalence in 13 year olds to 14 year olds in developing

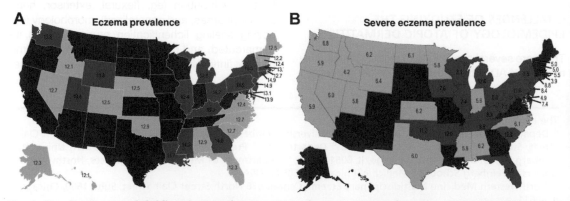

Fig. 1. The distribution of childhood AD and severe AD in the United States from the 2007–2008 NSCH. (A) AD prevalence (%); (B) severe AD prevalence (%). Data were divided into tertiles and color coded: tertile 1 = blue, tertile 2 = green, and tertile 3 = red.

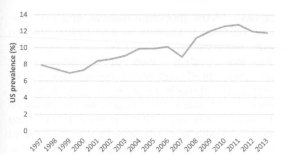

Fig. 2. The increasing prevalence of childhood AD (%) in the United States between 1997 and 2013 from the NHIS.

EPIDEMIOLOGY OF ADULT ATOPIC DERMATITIS

The conventional dogma has been that AD is a disorder of childhood, with few adults having active disease. Several recent studies suggest, however, that AD may be more common in adults than previously recognized. International studies of AD in adults found prevalence ranging from 2.0% to 6.9% prior to 2000 depending on regional and methodological differences.[26-30] Recent studies, however, of 27,157 and 34,613 adults (ages 18–85 years) from the 2010 NHIS and 2012 NHIS found 1-year prevalence of AD in 10.2% and 7.2%, respectively.[31,32] Both of these studies randomly sampled adults from nationally representative cohorts from all 50 states and assessed for self-reported disease using an in-person survey. The 2010 NHIS used a less specific question about "dermatitis, eczema, or any other red, inflamed skin rash,"[32] which overestimates the disease prevalence. In contrast, the 2012 NHIS used a more specific question about "eczema or skin allergy,"[31] which was similar to the previously validated question used in the NSCH but not a health care diagnosis. In the 2012 NHIS, the prevalence of AD peaked in early childhood (14%), remained high throughout childhood (13%–14%), decreased somewhat during adolescence (8%), and then remained stable throughout adulthood (6%–8%) (Fig. 3).

There are several possible explanations for the higher-than-expected prevalence of AD in adults. First, AD may not burn out, or dissipate, as much as previously thought. A study of the 7157 children from the Pediatric Eczema Elective Registry, a phase 4 registry of topical pimecrolimus users, found that at every age, more than 80% of subjects had symptoms of AD and/or were using medication to treat their AD.[33] It was not until

nations.[9] Consistent with the previously mentioned studies in the United States, the ISAAC study along with other smaller population-based and/or community-based studies suggest higher AD prevalence in wealthier, developed nations compared with poorer, developing nations.[3,8,10-18] Caution is required when interpreting prevalence estimates in some countries, for example, Ethiopia, where the ISAAC definition of AD did not perform well.[19,20] A systematic review of 69 studies examining international trends in AD between 1990 and 2010 demonstrated childhood AD prevalence rates greater than 20% in some developed nations, with increasing rates of AD in Africa, eastern Asia, western Europe, and parts of northern Europe.[21]

A UK study also demonstrated racial/ethnic disparities, in that London-born black children of Caribbean descent had a higher prevalence of AD than white children.[22] Some international studies demonstrated higher AD prevalence in advantaged socioeconomic groups,[23,24] whereas others did not[25] Several international studies found a slight female preponderance of AD,[8,16] whereas others found no associations between gender and AD.[3,7,11]

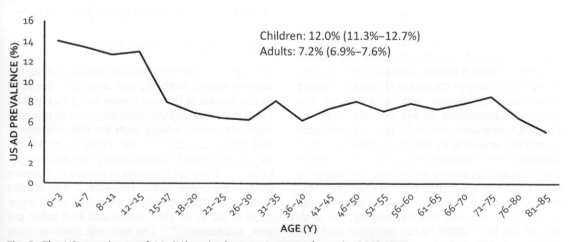

Children: 12.0% (11.3%–12.7%)
Adults: 7.2% (6.9%–7.6%)

Fig. 3. The US prevalence of AD (%) varies by age. Data are from the 2012 NHIS.

age 20 years that 50% of patients had at least 1 lifetime 6-month symptom-free and treatment-free period.[33] This cohort comprised, however, children from mostly urban locations, some with already longstanding disease, who received treatment of their AD by a health care provider with a nonsteroidal prescription topical agent, all of which may not be generalizable to the entire population. A recent systematic review of 46 studies (mostly birth cohorts) found a higher proportion of children with AD achieving an episode of clear skin (80% in 8 years).[34] Moreover, children whose AD started later in childhood or adolescence, was more severe, or already persistent for many years were less likely to achieve an episode of disease clearance.[34] It is likely that some of the children with an episode of clear skin had recurrent disease afterward. Thus, the overall persistence of childhood AD may be even higher.

Second, adult-onset AD may occur more commonly than previously thought. A US population-based study of 60,000 households found that 54% of respondents with empirically defined AD reported disease onset in adulthood.[2] Moreover, a retrospective Turkish study of 376 patients with AD found that 16.8% reported adult onset.[35] The issue of adult-onset AD is a little controversial, because some investigators might suggest that such patients may have had childhood disease but were unaware of it. Regardless of whether such cases are adult onset per se or adult recurrence, there seems a larger subset of patients with activation of their skin disease in adulthood than previously recognized.

Finally, it may be that the prevalence of AD has increased in adults over the years, similar to increases observed in children. This point has not been well studied to date and warrants further investigation.

ATOPIC DERMATITIS SEVERITY

AD severity assessments reflect a combination of symptoms (eg, itch and sleep disturbance), lesional severity (redness, thickness, lichenification, scaling, and so forth), and/or the extent of disease. Recent international consensus was achieved for the objective assessment of AD severity, with the Eczema Area and Severity Index and Scoring Atopic Dermatitis emerging as preferred assessments.[36] Although these assessments are routinely used in clinical trials or smaller-scale studies, they are rarely if ever used in a population-based setting. Thus, most studies of AD severity relied on self-reported or caregiver-reported disease severity. An analysis of the 2007–2008 NSCH demonstrated that 67.0% of US children had reportedly mild

disease, 26.0% moderate disease, and 7.0% severe disease, amounting to 2.98 million children with moderate-severe disease, with significant statewide variation[4,6] (see **Fig.** 1B). Although the prevalence of AD decreased with age, the relative proportions of moderate (ages 0–11 years: 24.7%; ages 12–17 years: 29.1%) and severe (ages 0–11 years: 6.7%; ages 12–17 years: 8.4%) disease increased with age. AD severity was also found worse in African Americans/blacks and Hispanics.[4,6] Other studies also suggested that African Americans/blacks may be prone to more severe disease[37,38] and increased health care utilization for AD[39] compared with whites. A population-based study of 1760 children living around Nottingham, England, found that 84% had mild, 14% moderate, and 2% severe disease as judged by a dermatologist.[40]

A household survey of 42,249 children and adults in 1998 found that 30% reported mild, 53% moderate, and 18% severe AD.[2] The high percentage of moderate-severe AD in this study may be due to selection bias. That is, patients with moderate-severe disease may have participated at higher rates than those with mild AD. Unfortunately, the study did not distinguish between pediatric versus adult patients.

Few population-based studies have directly assessed the prevalence of and risk factors for moderate-severe AD in adults. The 2013 National Health and Wellness Survey found that 50% of respondents with AD reported having moderate-severe disease.[41] The question used to assess for AD was not previously validated, however, and likely not sensitive enough, thereby missing many cases of AD. There was also a 15% nonresponse rate to the question about AD severity, raising concern for nonresponse bias. More population-based studies are needed to determine the prevalence and risk factors of moderate-severe AD in adults from the United States and internationally.

COST OF ATOPIC DERMATITIS

Although AD is typically nonfatal, there is substantial disease-related morbidity and disability. The 2010 Global Burden of Disease survey found that AD had the highest disability-adjusted life-years among skin disorders, which reflects both the high prevalence and patient burden.[42,43] The payer costs for AD vary by region and different health care delivery systems.[44,45] There are no recent estimates of the costs of AD in the United States. However, 2 older studies published in 1993 and 2002 estimated direct payer costs of AD to be $364 million and $3.8 billion per year, respectively.[46,47] This estimate, however, likely grossly underestimates the actual costs of the disease for several reasons. First, there has been considerable population growth globally. Second, the prevalence of AD has considerably increased since those periods of analysis, as discussed previously. Third, these estimates do not include costs associated with comorbid diseases or indirect costs. The patient burden of disease relates directly to the physical signs and symptoms of disease (eg, pruritus and pain) as well as indirectly to the harmful impact of skin symptoms on sleep (eg, difficulty falling asleep, more frequent awakenings, prolonged awakenings, and fragmented sleep),[31,48,49] mental health,[50–52] concentration, physical activity and sedentary behavior,[53] activities of daily living,[48] performance at school and work, increased sick days and missed days of work,[54] and so forth. Moreover, recent studies found significantly higher rates of multiple medical and mental health comorbidities in both children and adults with AD, including asthma, hay fever, food allergy,[4] alopecia areata,[55] cutaneous and extracutaneous infections,[56,57] depression,[51,52,58] anxiety,[58] attention-deficit/hyperactivity disorder,[50,58] osteoporosis,[59,60] fractures and other injuries,[59,61] anemia,[50] obesity,[62–67] cardiovascular risk factors,[64] and cardiovascular disease.[68] Most studies of the burden and cost of AD address the direct effects of the disease but not these myriad indirect effects and comorbidities.

Finally, studies of the payer costs of AD do not account for the immense patient costs in AD, secondary to increased health care utilization, copays, costs of over-the-counter emollients and medications, and so forth. A community survey found excess monthly out-of-pocket expenses of $9.94 for emollients and $7.88 for over-the-counter medications, totaling $213 annually per patient.[69] A recent questionnaire-based study of AD patients (or parents) from an academic medical center found excess costs of $274 in the preceding month, with $75 from direct costs and $199 from indirect costs.[70] Two US population studies found excess out-of-pocket costs related to health care utilization of $$371 to $489 per person-year in adults with AD.[54] Thus, the economic burden of AD is likely much greater than previously reported direct payer costs.

SUMMARY

In conclusion, AD poses a considerable public health burden owing to its high prevalence in both children and adults, high proportion of patients with moderate and severe disease, disease-related disability, and higher direct and indirect costs to payers and patients alike. Future research is needed to identify population-based risk factors and opportunities for disease prevention.

REFERENCES

1. Kantor R, Thyssen JP, Paller AS, et al. Atopic dermatitis, atopic eczema, or eczema? A systematic review, meta-analysis, and recommendation for uniform use of 'atopic dermatitis'. Allergy 2016;71(10):1480–5.
2. Hanifin JM, Reed ML, Eczema P, et al. A population-based survey of eczema prevalence in the United States. Dermatitis 2007;18(2):82–91.
3. Shaw TE, Currie GP, Koudelka CW, et al. Eczema prevalence in the United States: data from the 2003 National Survey of Children's Health. J Invest Dermatol 2011;131(1):67–73.
4. Silverberg JI, Simpson EL. Association between severe eczema in children and multiple comorbid conditions and increased healthcare utilization. Pediatr Allergy Immunol 2013;24(5):476–86.
5. Silverberg JI, Patel N, Immaneni S, et al. Assessment of atopic dermatitis using self-report and caregiver report: a multicentre validation study. Br J Dermatol 2015;173(6):1400–4.
6. Silverberg JI, Simpson EL. Associations of childhood eczema severity: a US population-based study. Dermatitis 2014;25(3):107–14.
7. Silverberg JI, Hanifin J, Simpson EL. Climatic factors are associated with childhood eczema prevalence in the United States. J Invest Dermatol 2013;133(7): 1752–9.
8. Odhiambo JA, Williams HC, Clayton TO, et al. Global variations in prevalence of eczema symptoms in children from ISAAC phase three. J Allergy Clin Immunol 2009;124(6):1251–8.e23.
9. Williams H, Stewart A, von Mutius E, et al. Is eczema really on the increase worldwide? J Allergy Clin Immunol 2008;121(4):947–54.e15.
10. Purvis DJ, Thompson JM, Clark PM, et al. Risk factors for atopic dermatitis in New Zealand children at 3.5 years of age. Br J Dermatol 2005;152(4):742–9.
11. Tay YK, Kong KH, Khoo L, et al. The prevalence and descriptive epidemiology of atopic dermatitis in Singapore school children. Br J Dermatol 2002; 146(1):101–6.
12. Martin PE, Koplin JJ, Eckert JK, et al. The prevalence and socio-demographic risk factors of clinical eczema in infancy: a population-based observational study. Clin Exp Allergy 2013;43(6):642–51.
13. Xu F, Yan S, Li F, et al. Prevalence of childhood atopic dermatitis: an urban and rural community-based study in Shanghai, China. PLoS One 2012; 7(5):e36174.
14. Belyhun Y, Amberbir A, Medhin G, et al. Prevalence and risk factors of wheeze and eczema in 1-year-old children: the Butajira birth cohort, Ethiopia. Clin Exp Allergy 2010;40(4):619–26.
15. Kay J, Gawkrodger DJ, Mortimer MJ, et al. The prevalence of childhood atopic eczema in a general population. J Am Acad Dermatol 1994;30(1):35–9.

16. Schultz Larsen F, Diepgen T, Svensson A. The occurrence of atopic dermatitis in north Europe: an international questionnaire study. J Am Acad Dermatol 1996;34(5 Pt 1):760–4.

17. Sugiura H, Umemoto N, Deguchi H, et al. Prevalence of childhood and adolescent atopic dermatitis in a Japanese population: comparison with the disease frequency examined 20 years ago. Acta Derm Venereol 1998;78(4):293–4.

18. Kanwar AJ, De D. Epidemiology and clinical features of atopic dermatitis in India. Indian J Dermatol 2011;56(5):471–5.

19. Haileamlak A, Lewis SA, Britton J, et al. Validation of the International Study of Asthma and Allergies in Children (ISAAC) and U.K. criteria for atopic eczema in Ethiopian children. Br J Dermatol 2005;152(4):735–41.

20. Oien T, Storro O, Johnsen R. Assessing atopic disease in children two to six years old: reliability of a revised questionnaire. Prim Care Respir J 2008;17(3):164–8.

21. Deckers IA, McLean S, Linssen S, et al. Investigating international time trends in the incidence and prevalence of atopic eczema 1990-2010: a systematic review of epidemiological studies. PloS one 2012;7(7):e39803.

22. Williams HC, Pembroke AC, Forsdyke H, et al. London-born black Caribbean children are at increased risk of atopic dermatitis. J Am Acad Dermatol 1995;32(2 Pt 1):212–7.

23. Williams HC, Strachan DP, Hay RJ. Childhood eczema: disease of the advantaged? BMJ 1994;308(6937):1132–5.

24. Taylor-Robinson DC, Williams H, Pearce A, et al. Do early-life exposures explain why more advantaged children get eczema? Findings from the U.K. Millennium Cohort Study. Br J Dermatol 2016;174(3):569–78.

25. Mercer MJ, Joubert G, Ehrlich RI, et al. Socioeconomic status and prevalence of allergic rhinitis and atopic eczema symptoms in young adolescents. Pediatr Allergy Immunol 2004;15(3):234–41.

26. Muto T, Hsieh SD, Sakurai Y, et al. Prevalence of atopic dermatitis in Japanese adults. Br J Dermatol 2003;148(1):117–21.

27. Saeki H, Tsunemi Y, Fujita H, et al. Prevalence of atopic dermatitis determined by clinical examination in Japanese adults. J Dermatol 2006;33(11):817–9.

28. Marks R, Kilkenny M, Plunkett A, et al. The prevalence of common skin conditions in Australian school students: 2. Atopic dermatitis. Br J Dermatol 1999;140(3):468–73.

29. Dotterud LK, Falk ES. Atopic disease among adults in Northern Russia, an area with heavy air pollution. Acta Derm Venereol 1999;79(6):448–50.

30. Herd RM, Tidman MJ, Prescott RJ, et al. Prevalence of atopic eczema in the community: the Lothian Atopic Dermatitis study. Br J Dermatol 1996;135(1):18–9.

31. Silverberg JI, Garg NK, Paller AS, et al. Sleep disturbances in adults with eczema are associated with impaired overall health: a US population-based study. J Invest Dermatol 2015;135(1):56–66.

32. Silverberg JI, Hanifin JM. Adult eczema prevalence and associations with asthma and other health and demographic factors: a US population-based study. J Allergy Clin Immunol 2013;132(5):1132–8.

33. Margolis JS, Abuabara K, Bilker W, et al. Persistence of mild to moderate atopic dermatitis. JAMA Dermatol 2014;150(6):593–600.

34. Kim JP, Chao LX, Simpson EL, et al. Persistence of atopic dermatitis (AD): a systematic review and meta-analysis. J Am Acad Dermatol 2016;75(4):681–7.e11.

35. Ozkaya E. Adult-onset atopic dermatitis. J Am Acad Dermatol 2005;52(4):579–82.

36. Chalmers JR, Schmitt J, Apfelbacher C, et al. Report from the third international consensus meeting to harmonise core outcome measures for atopic eczema/dermatitis clinical trials (HOME). Br J Dermatol 2014;171(6):1318–25.

37. Vachiramon V, Tey HL, Thompson AE, et al. Atopic dermatitis in African American children: addressing unmet needs of a common disease. Pediatr Dermatol 2012;29(4):395–402.

38. Ben-Gashir MA, Hay RJ. Reliance on erythema scores may mask severe atopic dermatitis in black children compared with their white counterparts. Br J Dermatol 2002;147(5):920–5.

39. Horii KA, Simon SD, Liu DY, et al. Atopic dermatitis in children in the United States, 1997-2004: visit trends, patient and provider characteristics, and prescribing patterns. Pediatrics 2007;120(3):e527–34.

40. Emerson RM, Williams HC, Allen BR. Severity distribution of atopic dermatitis in the community and its relationship to secondary referral. Br J Dermatol 1998;139(1):73–6.

41. Whiteley J, Emir B, Seitzman R, et al. The burden of atopic dermatitis in US adults: results from the 2013 National Health and Wellness Survey. Curr Med Res Opin 2016;21:1–7.

42. Murray CJ, Vos T, Lozano R, et al. Disability-adjusted life years (DALYs) for 291 diseases and injuries in 21 regions, 1990-2010: a systematic analysis for the Global Burden of Disease Study 2010. Lancet 2012;380(9859):2197–223.

43. Vos T, Flaxman AD, Naghavi M, et al. Years lived with disability (YLDs) for 1160 sequelae of 289 diseases and injuries 1990-2010: a systematic analysis for the Global Burden of Disease Study 2010. Lancet 2012;380(9859):2163–96.

44. Mancini AJ, Kaulback K, Chamlin SL. The socioeconomic impact of atopic dermatitis in the United States: a systematic review. Pediatr Dermatol 2008;25(1):1–6.

45. Verboom P, Hakkaart-Van L, Sturkenboom M, et al. The cost of atopic dermatitis in the Netherlands: an

international comparison. Br J Dermatol 2002;147(4): 716–24.

46. Ellis CN, Drake LA, Prendergast MM, et al. Cost of atopic dermatitis and eczema in the United States. J Am Acad Dermatol 2002;46(3):361–70.

47. Lapidus CS, Schwarz DF, Honig PJ. Atopic dermatitis in children: who cares? Who pays? J Am Acad Dermatol 1993;28(5 Pt 1):699–703.

48. Yu SH, Attarian H, Zee P, et al. Burden of sleep and fatigue in US adults with atopic dermatitis. Dermatitis 2016;27(2):50–8.

49. Fishbein AB, Vitaterna O, Haugh IM, et al. Nocturnal eczema: review of sleep and circadian rhythms in children with atopic dermatitis and future research directions. J Allergy Clin Immunol 2015;136(5):1170–7.

50. Strom MA, Fishbein AB, Paller AS, et al. Association between atopic dermatitis and attention deficit hyperactivity disorder in U.S. children and adults. Br J Dermatol 2016;175(5):920–9.

51. Yu SH, Silverberg JI. Association between atopic dermatitis and depression in US Adults. J Invest Dermatol 2015;135(12):3183–6.

52. Garg N, Silverberg JI. Association between childhood allergic disease, psychological comorbidity, and injury requiring medical attention. Ann Allergy Asthma Immunol 2014;112(6):525–32.

53. Strom MA, Silverberg JI. Associations of physical activity and sedentary behavior with atopic disease in United States children. J Pediatr 2016; 174:247–53.e3.

54. Silverberg JI. Health care utilization, patient costs, and access to care in US adults with eczema: a population-based study. JAMA Dermatol 2015; 151(7):743–52.

55. Mohan GC, Silverberg JI. Association of vitiligo and alopecia areata with atopic dermatitis: a systematic review and meta-analysis. JAMA Dermatol 2015; 151(5):522–8.

56. Silverberg JI, Silverberg NB. Childhood atopic dermatitis and warts are associated with increased risk of infection: a US population-based study. J Allergy Clin Immunol 2014;133(4):1041–7.

57. Strom MA, Silverberg JI. Association between atopic dermatitis and extracutaneous infections in US adults. Br J Dermatol 2016;176(2):495–7.

58. Yaghmaie P, Koudelka CW, Simpson EL. Mental health comorbidity in patients with atopic dermatitis. J Allergy Clin Immunol 2013;131(2):428–33.

59. Garg NK, Silverberg JI. Eczema is associated with osteoporosis and fractures in adults: a US population-based study. J Allergy Clin Immunol 2015;135(4):1085–7.e2.

60. Silverberg JI. Association between childhood atopic dermatitis, malnutrition and low bone mineral density: a US population based study. Pediatr Allergy Immunol 2015;26(1):54–61.

61. Garg N, Silverberg JI. Association between eczema and increased fracture and bone or joint injury in adults: a US population-based study. JAMA Dermatol 2015;151(1):33–41.

62. Silverberg JI. Role of childhood obesity in atopic dermatitis. Exper Rev Dermatol 2011;6(6):635–42.

63. Silverberg JI, Becker L, Kwasny M, et al. Central obesity and high blood pressure in pediatric patients with atopic dermatitis. JAMA Dermatol 2015; 151(2):144–52.

64. Silverberg JI, Greenland P. Eczema and cardiovascular risk factors in 2 US adult population studies. J Allergy Clin Immunol 2015;135(3):721–8.e6.

65. Silverberg JI, Kleiman E, Lev-Tov H, et al. Association between obesity and atopic dermatitis in childhood: a case-control study. J Allergy Clin Immunol 2011;127(5):1180–6.e1.

66. Silverberg JI, Silverberg NB, Lee-Wong M. Association between atopic dermatitis and obesity in adulthood. Br J Dermatol 2012;166(3):498–504.

67. Zhang A, Silverberg JI. Association of atopic dermatitis with overweight and obesity: a systematic review and meta-analysis. J Am Acad Dermatol 2015;72(4): 606–16.e4.

68. Silverberg JI. Association between adult atopic dermatitis, cardiovascular disease, and increased heart attacks in three population-based studies. Allergy 2015;70(10):1300–8.

69. Anderson RT, Rajagopalan R. Effects of allergic dermatosis on health-related quality of life. Curr Allergy Asthma Rep 2001;1(4):309–15.

70. Filanovsky MG, Pootongkam S, Tamburro JE, et al. The financial and emotional impact of atopic dermatitis on children and their families. J Pediatr 2016; 169:284–90.e5.

The Long-Term Course of Atopic Dermatitis

Katrina Abuabara, MD, MA, MSCE[a],[*], David J. Margolis, MD, PhD[b],
Sinéad M. Langan, FRCP, MSc, PhD[c],[d]

KEYWORDS

- Atopic dermatitis • Eczema • Atopic eczema • Epidemiology • Natural history • Clinical course

KEY POINTS

- Atopic dermatitis (AD) is a chronic, relapsing condition, meaning that the intensity of symptoms usually fluctuates over time.
- Changes in skin physiology may be evident from birth, suggesting that AD may be a lifelong condition marked by intermittent symptoms/disease activity.
- Because AD is episodic, AD incidence, prevalence, persistence, remission, flare, and long-term control require careful definition.
- Improved measurement of the frequency and duration of active disease periods can help to elucidate more about the clinical course AD and the role of treatment in long-term outcomes.

INTRODUCTION

Atopic dermatitis (AD) (also known as atopic eczema or eczema) is by definition a chronic condition. The original diagnostic criteria proposed by Hanifin and Rajka and the most recent guidelines issued by the American Academy of Dermatology both include a "chronic or relapsing" history as an essential feature.[1,2] Little is written, however, about the clinical course of AD.[3] This could be because many patients with AD present with symptoms early in life, and hence most research has focused on pediatric disease. Although there are relatively few publications about adult disease, recent population-based estimates of AD prevalence among US children and adults were similar.[4–6] These data suggest either AD begins in childhood and persists through adulthood, childhood AD remits for some and begins in adulthood for others, or some combination thereof. A number of practical and methodological challenges to studying a chronic episodic condition have limited the description of the long-term course of AD. In the following sections, we review the available data and discuss the implications for clinical care and future research.

WHY IS THE LONG-TERM COURSE OF ATOPIC DERMATITIS IMPORTANT TO STUDY?

Data about the long-term course of AD are necessary for informing clinicians and patients about prognosis and guiding treatment decisions at an individual level and for planning at the health systems level. Traditionally, AD was considered a pediatric condition and families were told most children "outgrow" AD by adolescence. Such imprecise information is insufficient for patients

Disclosure Statement: The authors have nothing to disclose.
[a] Department of Dermatology, University of California San Francisco (UCSF), 2340 Sutter Street, N421, San Francisco, CA 94115, USA; [b] Faculty of Epidemiology and Population Health, London School of Hygiene and Tropical Medicine, Keppel St, Bloomsbury, London WC1E 7HT, UK; [c] Department of Dermatology, University of Pennsylvania Perelman School of Medicine, 3400 Civic Center Boulevard, Philadelphia, PA 19104, USA; [d] Department of Biostatistics and Epidemiology, University of Pennsylvania Perelman School of Medicine, 3400 Civic Center Boulevard, Philadelphia, PA 19104, USA
* Corresponding author.
E-mail address: katrina.abuabara@ucsf.edu

Dermatol Clin 35 (2017) 291–297
http://dx.doi.org/10.1016/j.det.2017.02.003
0733-8635/17/Crown Copyright © 2017 Published by Elsevier Inc. All rights reserved.

who desire detailed prognostic data. Moreover, it is insufficient for understanding the impact of potentially disease-modifying interventions, a topic of particular salience in the current era of systemic drug development.

WHEN DOES ATOPIC DERMATITIS BEGIN?

The symptoms of AD may begin at any age, although many sources suggest that most incident AD occurs in early childhood. Estimates may be affected by study designs that focus only on pediatric or clinic populations or by the diagnostic criteria used. For example, a recent review in the *Lancet* states "in roughly 60% of cases, the disease manifests during the first year of life," citing a prospective study that follows patients until age 7 and a retrospective cohort of clinic patients.[7–9] Studies including only children may underestimate the average age of disease onset because they would not capture adult-onset cases. Similarly, clinic-based samples are likely biased toward patients with more persistent or severe disease that begins earlier in life, and may not be not be representative of the general AD population. Additionally, some commonly used diagnostic criteria, including the Hanifin and Rajka criteria[2] and the UK Working Party criteria,[10] include onset in childhood as a minor criterion. Studies using these criteria may estimate lower rates of adult disease compared with studies that do not select patients based on age of onset. Data that are less likely to be susceptible to selection bias suggest that AD may commonly begin in adulthood. For example, a population-based survey in the United States found that 54% of those with AD reported disease onset after age 18.[11] More data are needed to understand disease incidence over the life span and whether adult-onset disease is different from disease that begins in childhood.

DOES ATOPIC DERMATITIS PERMANENTLY RESOLVE, AND IF SO, WHEN?

Existing data are unable to answer this question. An older review found that 50% to 70% of individuals with AD improved over 10 years of follow-up, although the definition of clearance varied by study and ranged from 11% to 92%.[3] Population-based birth cohort studies with multiple assessments of individuals over 2 decades found that rates of "short-term" or "apparent" clearance decreased when accounting for subsequent recurrences using estimates of annual period prevalence repeated every 3 to 7 years.[12–15] More frequent measurement of disease activity every 6 months in a US cohort of children and young adults with AD who had prior treatment with a topical calcineurin

inhibitor (and therefore may be more likely to have persistent disease) suggests that although some patients seem to improve with age, most continue to have active disease at multiple time points.[16] Longitudinal studies that follow individuals throughout adulthood are needed to better understand the periodicity of disease activity and patterns over the life course.

IS ATOPIC DERMATITIS A LIFELONG CONDITION?

Genetic and physiologic data support the idea of AD as a lifelong condition. It is well established that AD runs in families, and in the past decade genetic discoveries have implicated multiple genes involved in the development and maintenance of the skin barrier and immune function.[17,18] Patients with AD often have xerosis that predates their diagnosis. In fact, "a history of generally dry skin from birth" was found to be one of the most predictive characteristics and hence was included among the minimum set of discriminators in the UK Working Party diagnostic criteria.[10] Although the evidence is mixed,[19] some studies have shown that physiologic differences, such as transepidermal water loss (TEWL), may precede the clinical manifestations of AD and are detectable as early as day 2 after birth.[20,21] Moreover, experimental evidence from 2 randomized trials suggest that maintenance of the skin barrier with emollients during the neonatal period may delay or prevent the development of clinical signs of AD.[22,23]

These data suggest that individuals with AD have an elevated probability of developing clinical symptoms throughout life, as illustrated in **Fig. 1**. Even normal-appearing skin in patients with AD has evidence of differences in skin barrier function, dendritic cell population, and cytokine profiles, supporting the concept of subclinical disease.[24] The factors influencing the transition to clinically

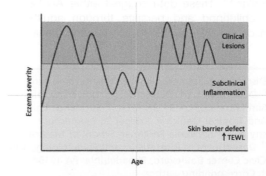

Fig. 1. Hypothetical example illustrating the long-term course of AD.

evident disease (both disease onset and disease flares) are an area of active research: investigators have explored the modulation of immune priming by hygiene, environmental factors, psychosocial factors, and diet.[25–27] Early disease onset, severe early disease, family history of atopic disease, female sex, low income, black race, and filaggrin mutations have all been associated with more active or prolonged disease.[3,28–30] Recent data also suggest the skin microbiome appears to be different in both lesional and nonlesional skin between young children and teenagers/adults with AD.[31] There is little consensus, however, about the causes of disease onset or progression, and there are few studies examining factors that result in long-term or permanent disease remission.

Some investigators have suggested that there may be phases through which individuals are likely to pass, including the development of "autosensitization" and eventually, chronic "autoimmune" disease.[32] Whether eczema predisposes to asthma and allergies, a phenomenon termed the "atopic march," is also a matter of active debate.[33,34] Furthermore, it is unclear whether treatment of AD might affect the long-term clinical course or prevent the development of comorbid conditions, although there is some limited evidence to suggest that good control of eczema may have beneficial effects on respiratory disease as well.[32] More data are needed to understand whether the onset and persistence of AD symptoms are part of a causal pathway to progressive disease, or whether barrier and immune dysfunction are always present and symptoms simply emerge when an individual encounters triggers throughout life.

CHALLENGES TO STUDYING THE LONG-TERM COURSE OF ATOPIC DERMATITIS

The chronic and episodic nature of AD renders it particularly challenging to study. We discuss epidemiologic concepts and their application to AD in the following sections and in **Table 1**.

Incidence

Incidence refers to the rate of new cases of a disease over a specified period; however, AD may be difficult to diagnose very early in its course because its presentation is clinically heterogeneous. Diagnostic criteria for AD often include a measure of chronicity, complicating the decision of when to define an incident case. A systematic review of prevention studies found that in practice, there is a large degree of variability in the methods used to define an incident case of AD, and 27% of studies did not report any definition at all.[35] The investigators propose a modification to the UK Working Party criteria for AD that requires a history of an itchy skin condition that is either continuous or is intermittent for at least 4 weeks. Longitudinal cohort studies that examine AD should be careful to explicitly state how the date of onset is defined and to ensure that their methods do not introduce immortal time bias.

Prevalence

Prevalence is typically defined as the proportion of a population with the condition of interest. Many individuals with AD have periods during which they may have no visible skin lesions and/or bothersome symptoms. For conditions that are intermittent, a point prevalence based on a single

---

Table 1
Methodological considerations for studying the long-term course of atopic dermatitis

Concept	Considerations	Recommendations
Incidence	Must be chronic to meet most diagnostic criteria	Specify minimum duration of symptoms required for diagnosis (4 weeks has been proposed)[34]
Prevalence	Dependent on time period and definition	Specify method of ascertainment (ie, physical examination vs self-report) and definition used
Remission/Persistence	Dependent on length of follow-up and method of detection	Avoid using these terms; specify age of patient and duration of follow-up without treatment and/or symptoms
Flare	Dependent on patient's baseline; difficult to ascertain exact duration	Clearly define; delineate disease activity from disease severity; consider combination of a patient-reported outcome and a severity score or behavioral measure such as 'escalation of treatment'
Long-term control	No consensus on measurement	Clearly define; consider use of well-controlled weeks[45]

examination may underestimate the condition's frequency. Therefore, a period prevalence, defined as the proportion of cases within a specified time frame, is often preferred. The ISAAC studies found self-reported annual period prevalence was 2 to 3 times higher than prevalence based on physical examination in many settings.[36]

The duration of symptom-free periods among patients with AD is poorly understood and therefore it is unclear what frequency of assessment is necessary to capture those with intermittent disease. Some studies report lifetime prevalence, although such estimates should be interpreted with caution based on the age of the sample and method of reporting. Studies of older patients may be prone to recall bias (ie, they may not remember disease that was active only in early life), whereas studies of younger patients will miss those with adult-onset disease. Moreover, given the increase in awareness of allergic diseases over the past few decades, there is the possibility for increased reporting over time, especially of more mild cases.

Remission and Persistence

Conditions such as cancer are considered to be "in remission" when they become undetectable. This concept has been applied to AD, but we warrant caution in the use of this term given the episodic nature of the condition and complexities of defining inactive disease. In AD, there are many ways inactive disease might be defined, including normal skin appearance, cessation of symptoms, such as itch, discontinuation of treatment, and biomarkers or tests of barrier function. It is unclear at present what the optimal approach to defining AD remission is, and whether there is a minimum period during which AD must be undetectable for remission to be defined. Some individuals may have recurrence of skin lesions after decades without disease.

Long periods of latency add confusion around the distinction between AD and other types of dermatitis in adults. Patients with AD have both disrupted barrier and immune mechanisms that may potentiate them toward increased rates of allergic and irritant contact dermatitis, and it may be difficult to differentiate these conditions from AD disease activity.[37,38]

Many studies refer to disease "persistence"; yet few define what is meant by this term.[39] Often, persistence is used to refer to whether patients who are followed longitudinally report symptoms at subsequent follow-up, a definition that is highly dependent on the selection of the cohort, timing of follow-up, and measure of disease activity. Ideally, a readily measurable

biomarker would enable prediction of lesion and symptom recurrence, although attempts to date have not elucidated useful biomarkers for either diagnosis or prognosis.[40] Until better prospective data with clear markers of disease activity that can be used to define "remission" and "persistence" are available, we recommend that investigators avoid using these terms and instead clearly define what is being measured.

Flare

Although the term "flare" is commonly used to refer to disease worsening or exacerbation, many studies define flares differently.[41,42] A recent systematic review highlighted that among 26 studies incorporating AD flares as outcome measures, 21 different definitions were used and only 4 studies incorporated a patient-reported outcome. Three broad approaches have been used by investigators to define AD flares: arbitrary cutoffs on severity scales, composite measures (including symptoms and signs of AD), and behavioral approaches (such as use of treatments). The challenges with these approaches are varied. First, using an arbitrary cutoff of an "objective" severity score may be attractive, as it potentially reduces information bias; however, it does so at the expense of not having a patient-reported outcome, and it also adds expense and logistic challenges because it requires physician review at short notice. Second, using a composite measure is appealing, as it includes multiple dimensions; however, interpreting the meaning of the flare definition may be difficult. For the behavioral approach, the advantages include being patient reported; however, there is considerable discussion in the eczema literature about avoidance of topical corticosteroid use, hence behavior may not totally capture disease activity.[43] A validation study found that "use of topical anti-inflammatory medications" and "escalation of treatment" were reasonable approaches to capturing flares, and that the former outcome was feasible to collect in longer-term studies.[42]

Given the variability of flare definitions, it is difficult to summarize patterns of disease activity. One estimate comes from the International Study of Life with Atopic Eczema (ISOLTE) trial that included 2000 patients with moderate-to-severe disease. The study found that patients spend, on average, 1 of 3 days in flare (average 9 flares per year lasting 15 days each time), with flare defined as a "sudden worsening of symptoms requiring a physician consultation or application of prescription medication."[44] This study included patients from 8 countries, but recruited individuals from physician's offices and therefore may not be representative of the average individual with AD.

MEASURES OF LONG-TERM CONTROL

Given the challenges inherent in studying a chronic episodic disease, how might future studies measure long-term disease control? A recent systematic review aiming to identify how long-term control was captured in published randomized controlled trials found little consistency and highlighted the need for standardized measures.[45] Methods included repeated measures of patient-reported or clinician-reported outcomes (such as severity, pruritus, sleep quality of life, affected body surface area, or global assessment scores), changes in medication use, and flares. Time to next disease exacerbation or number of disease flares have been proposed, but depend on clear delineation of the start and end of a flare and may require frequent measurement. The number of totally and well-controlled weeks has also been recommended as a possible approach to assessing long-term control in AD.[46] Defining long-term control in AD is recommended as a core outcome domain for clinical studies of AD, but there is currently no widely accepted or validated approach to defining this outcome.[3] The Harmonizing Outcome Measures in Eczema initiative has prioritized this topic as a focus for their 2017 consensus meeting.

LONG-TERM TREATMENT

Management approaches should address the intermittent and chronic nature of AD. Much research has focused on "reactive" approaches that treat disease flares or periods of acute worsening. Newer guidelines emphasize the role of "proactive" approaches with continued use of either topical corticosteroids (1–2 times per week) or topical calcineurin inhibitors (2–3 times per week) after disease stabilization to reduce subsequent flares or relapses.[1] Structured education programs and avoidance if there is evidence of a true immunoglobulin E–mediated allergy are also recommended based on the highest level of evidence. Gaps in research include comparative studies to decide on the best agents for long-term maintenance therapy, long-term safety data for intermittent use of topical steroids and calcineurin inhibitors, and high-quality evidence for the long-term use of systemic therapies in AD.[1,47] Additionally, a high priority for future research is to determine whether treatments may modify the clinical course and/or prevent the development of other allergic outcomes.

SUMMARY

The long-term course of AD is an important area for additional research. We have highlighted a number of methodological considerations that warrant careful attention in study design and reporting. Defining the clinical course of AD provides the foundation for understanding the results of interventional studies and establishing whether new treatments might modify the course of disease. Moreover, an understanding of the long-term course of disease can help contextualize trial findings. If some patients are more likely to have persistent disease, trials should report the relevant baseline characteristics and consider prespecified subgroup analyses (such as initial age of disease onset, duration of active disease before baseline. In conclusion, understanding associations with the long-term course of disease would provide prognostic information for patients and help providers to design comprehensive treatment programs.

REFERENCES

1. Eichenfield LF, Tom WL, Chamlin SL, et al. Guidelines of care for the management of atopic dermatitis: section 1. Diagnosis and assessment of atopic dermatitis. J Am Acad Dermatol 2014;70(2):338–51.
2. Hanifin JM, Rajka G. Diagnostic features of atopic dermatitis. Acta Derm Venereol 1980;92(suppl): 44–7.
3. Williams HC, Wuthrich B. The natural history of atopic dermatitis. Atopic dermatitis: the epidemiology, causes and prevention of atopic eczema. Cambridge, United Kingdom: Cambridge University Press; 2000.
4. Abuabara K, Margolis DJ. Do children really outgrow their eczema, or is there more than one eczema? J Allergy Clin Immunol 2013;132(5):1139–40.
5. Silverberg JI, Hanifin JM. Adult eczema prevalence and associations with asthma and other health and demographic factors: a US population-based study. J Allergy Clin Immunol 2013; 132(5):1132–8.
6. Shaw TE, Currie GP, Koudelka CW, et al. Eczema prevalence in the United States: data from the 2003 National Survey of Children's Health. J Invest Dermatol 2011;131(1):67–73.
7. Weidinger S, Novak N. Atopic dermatitis. Lancet 2016;387(10023):1109–22.
8. Illi S, von Mutius E, Lau S, et al. The natural course of atopic dermatitis from birth to age 7 years and the association with asthma. J Allergy Clin Immunol 2004;113(5):925–31.
9. Garmhausen D, Hagemann T, Bieber T, et al. Characterization of different courses of atopic dermatitis

in adolescent and adult patients. Allergy 2013;68(4):498–506.

10. Williams HC, Burney PG, Hay RJ, et al. The U.K. working party's diagnostic criteria for atopic dermatitis. I. Derivation of a minimum set of discriminators for atopic dermatitis. Br J Dermatol 1994;131(3):383–96.

11. Hanifin JM, Reed ML, Eczema P, et al. A population-based survey of eczema prevalence in the United States. Dermatitis 2007;18(2):82–91.

12. Ballardini N, Kull I, Lind T, et al. Development and comorbidity of eczema, asthma and rhinitis to age 12: data from the BAMSE birth cohort. Allergy 2012;67(4):537–44.

13. Burr ML, Dunstan FD, Hand S, et al. The natural history of eczema from birth to adult life: a cohort study. Br J Dermatol 2013;168(6):1339–42.

14. Williams HC, Strachan DP. The natural history of childhood eczema: observations from the British 1958 birth cohort study. Br J Dermatol 1998;139(5):834–9.

15. Ziyab AH, Raza A, Karmaus W, et al. Trends in eczema in the first 18 years of life: results from the Isle of Wight 1989 birth cohort study. Clin Exp Allergy 2010;40(12):1776–84.

16. Abuabara K, Hoffstad O, Troxel A, et al. Atopic dermatitis disease control and age: a cohort study. J Allergy Clin Immunol 2015;136(1):190–2.e93.

17. Paternoster L, Standl M, Waage J, et al. Multi-ancestry genome-wide association study of 21,000 cases and 95,000 controls identifies new risk loci for atopic dermatitis. Nat Genet 2015;47(12):1449–56.

18. Elmose C, Thomsen SF. Twin studies of atopic dermatitis: interpretations and applications in the filaggrin era. J Allergy (Cairo) 2015;2015:902359.

19. Kikuchi K, Kobayashi H, O'Goshi K, et al. Impairment of skin barrier function is not inherent in atopic dermatitis patients: a prospective study conducted in newborns. Pediatr Dermatol 2006;23(2):109–13.

20. Kelleher M, Dunn-Galvin A, Hourihane JO, et al. Skin barrier dysfunction measured by transepidermal water loss at 2 days and 2 months predates and predicts atopic dermatitis at 1 year. J Allergy Clin Immunol 2015;135(4):930–5.e31.

21. Flohr C, England K, Radulovic S, et al. Filaggrin loss-of-function mutations are associated with early-onset eczema, eczema severity and transepidermal water loss at 3 months of age. Br J Dermatol 2010;163(6):1333–6.

22. Simpson EL, Chalmers JR, Hanifin JM, et al. Emollient enhancement of the skin barrier from birth offers effective atopic dermatitis prevention. J Allergy Clin Immunol 2014;134(4):818–23.

23. Horimukai K, Morita K, Narita M, et al. Application of moisturizer to neonates prevents development of atopic dermatitis. J Allergy Clin Immunol 2014;134(4):824–30.e26.

24. Tang TS, Bieber T, Williams HC. Are the concepts of induction of remission and treatment of subclinical inflammation in atopic dermatitis clinically useful? J Allergy Clin Immunol 2014;133(6):1615–25.e11.

25. Flohr C, Mann J. New insights into the epidemiology of childhood atopic dermatitis. Allergy 2014;69(1):3–16.

26. Langan SM, Bourke JF, Silcocks P, et al. An exploratory prospective observational study of environmental factors exacerbating atopic eczema in children. Br J Dermatol 2006;154(5):979–80.

27. Langan SM, Silcocks P, Williams HC. What causes flares of eczema in children? Br J Dermatol 2009;161(3):640–6.

28. Margolis DJ, Gupta J, Apter AJ, et al. Filaggrin-2 variation is associated with more persistent atopic dermatitis in African American subjects. J Allergy Clin Immunol 2014;133(3):784–9.

29. Margolis DJ, Apter AJ, Gupta J, et al. The persistence of atopic dermatitis and filaggrin (FLG) mutations in a US longitudinal cohort. J Allergy Clin Immunol 2012;130(4):912–7.

30. Margolis JS, Abuabara K, Bilker W, et al. Persistence of mild to moderate atopic dermatitis. JAMA Dermatol 2014;150(6):593–600.

31. Shi B, Bangayan NJ, Curd E, et al. The skin microbiome is different in pediatric versus adult atopic dermatitis. J Allergy Clin Immunol 2016;138(4):1233–6.

32. Bieber T, Cork M, Reitamo S. Atopic dermatitis: a candidate for disease-modifying strategy. Allergy 2012;67(8):969–75.

33. Bantz SK, Zhu Z, Zheng T. The atopic march: progression from atopic dermatitis to allergic rhinitis and asthma. J Clin Cell Immunol 2014;5(2):202.

34. Kapoor R, Menon C, Hoffstad O, et al. The prevalence of atopic triad in children with physician-confirmed atopic dermatitis. J Am Acad Dermatol 2008;58(1):68–73.

35. Simpson EL, Keck LE, Chalmers JR, et al. How should an incident case of atopic dermatitis be defined? A systematic review of primary prevention studies. J Allergy Clin Immunol 2012;130(1):137–44.

36. Flohr C, Weinmayr G, Weiland SK, et al. How well do questionnaires perform compared with physical examination in detecting flexural eczema? Findings from the International Study of Asthma and Allergies in Childhood (ISAAC) Phase Two. Br J Dermatol 2009;161(4):846–53.

37. Gittler JK, Krueger JG, Guttman-Yassky E. Atopic dermatitis results in intrinsic barrier and immune abnormalities: implications for contact dermatitis. J Allergy Clin Immunol 2013;131(2):300–13.

38. Mowad CM, Anderson B, Scheinman P, et al. Allergic contact dermatitis: patient diagnosis and evaluation. J Am Acad Dermatol 2016;74(6):1029–40.

39. Kim JP, Chao LX, Simpson EL, et al. Persistence of atopic dermatitis (AD): a systematic review and meta-analysis. J Am Acad Dermatol 2016;75(4): 681–7.e11.

40. Thijs J, Krastev T, Weidinger S, et al. Biomarkers for atopic dermatitis: a systematic review and meta-analysis. Curr Opin Allergy Clin Immunol 2015; 15(5):453–60.

41. Langan SM, Thomas KS, Williams HC. What is meant by a "flare" in atopic dermatitis? A systematic review and proposal. Arch Dermatol 2006;142(9):1190–6.

42. Thomas KS, Stuart B, O'Leary CJ, et al. Validation of treatment escalation as a definition of atopic eczema flares. PLoS One 2015;10(4):e0124770.

43. Charman CR, Morris AD, Williams HC. Topical corticosteroid phobia in patients with atopic eczema. Br J Dermatol 2000;142(5):931–6.

44. Zuberbier T, Orlow SJ, Paller AS, et al. Patient perspectives on the management of atopic dermatitis. J Allergy Clin Immunol 2006;118(1):226–32.

45. Barbarot S, Rogers NK, Abuabara K, et al. Strategies used for measuring long-term control in atopic dermatitis trials: a systematic review. J Am Acad Dermatol 2016;75(5):1038–44.

46. (HOME) HOMfE. Available at: http://www.nottingham. ac.uk/research/groups/cebd/resources/flare-atopic-dermatitis.aspx. Accessed October 1, 2016.

47. Ring J, Alomar A, Bieber T, et al. Guidelines for treatment of atopic eczema (atopic dermatitis) part II. J Eur Acad Dermatol Venereol 2012;26(9): 1176–93.

Adult-Onset Atopic Dermatitis: Fact or Fancy?

Jon M. Hanifin, MD

KEYWORDS

• Atopic dermatitis • Eczema • Topical therapy • Systemic therapy

KEY POINTS

- Atopic dermatitis (AD) therapy can be a challenge in many cases.
- Persistence into adulthood often reflects the more severe cases and such patients have the added problems of hand eczema and thick nummular lesions that resist topical medications.
- Within this group are patients labeled as having adult-onset AD, a designation that is hard to define and probably represents those whose childhood eczema was simply forgotten.
- Management is difficult for most adult cases and should not be diverted by questionable labels.

INTRODUCTION: DEFINING ADULT-ONSET ATOPIC DERMATITIS IS DIFFICULT

How is a reliable diagnosis conferred? Is it a distinct, exclusive phenotype? Do such patients relate to certain genotypes? It is known that, in general, AD begins in childhood, often infancy. Then it may regress in many or most instances, perhaps leaving only a few clues to its prior state, such as hand eczema, dry skin, lowered itch threshold, periods of flare with psychological stress, IgE-mediated allergies, infections, and season changes.

Interestingly, 4 decades ago, when gathering diagnostic indicators of AD,[1,2] most clinical focus revolved around adult cases, probably because they were more severe, thus persisting and finding their way to dermatologists. AD in children was generally much easier to control. Also, primary care physicians had typically been taught that AD was an allergic disease and the children were often referred to allergists.

With the recognition of distinctions between pediatric AD and adult AD (and perhaps the growth of the pediatric dermatology subspecialty), new attention was turned to criteria that applied to the range of infants, children, and adults. The advent of topical calcineurin inhibitors caused somewhat of a shift to new clinical approaches for childhood AD. Revised diagnostic guidelines,[3] more inclusive of children, appeared as a direct result of an American Academy of Dermatology meeting focused on topical calcineurin inhibitors, agents that were seen as possibly safer than topical corticosteroids (TCSs) for use in children. These advances helped promote the distinction between pediatric and adult eczemas and brought many more children into the offices of an increased range of practitioners. That in turn led to greater consciousness of dermatologists regarding adult forms of AD. The disease was always assumed to be characterized by onset in childhood. But many adults had no recollection of childhood eczema.

Increased awareness of the full spectrum of AD may have influenced the suggestion of adult-onset AD as a distinct entity, starting with an Australian report in 2000,[4] and subsequent reports have come from many sectors, including Italy,[5,6] Turkey,[7] Greece,[8] Taiwan,[9] and India.[10]

Unfortunately, there are no validated criteria for defining this category. Hence, new questions arise, including those that began this article. Some features help explain apparent onset of AD during adulthood (**Box 1**). Clear diagnosis of

Department of Dermatology, Oregon Health & Science University, 3303 Bond Avenue, Portland, OR 97239, USA
E-mail address: hanifinj@ohsu.edu

Dermatol Clin 35 (2017) 299–302
http://dx.doi.org/10.1016/j.det.2017.02.009
0733-8635/17/© 2017 Elsevier Inc. All rights reserved.

derm.theclinics.com

> **Box 1**
> **Features associated with claims of adult-onset atopic dermatitis**
>
> - Childhood spent in humid sunny or tropical climate
> - First AD diagnosis made only after change of residence to a cold dry climate or exposure to central heating
> - Onset of hand eczema after all other features of AD have regressed
> - Recurrence of AD after infection or other stressor

adult-onset AD requires absence of childhood history. Certainly, people spending childhood and adolescence in warm, sunny, humid regions might never have had diagnosable AD. That clearly is the situation with many of the patients who immigrate or study in the United States from Southeast Asia and South and Central America. Beyond the transition to drier climates, the trappings of first-world living, with central heating and overbathing, are likely another major stimulus for adult-onset AD among relocated individuals.

Conversely, for patients who have not made such transitions, it seems imprecise to make a diagnosis of adult-onset AD. Mild cases of previous childhood eczema are likely to be missed. Naleway and colleagues[11] reported a high rate of recall bias in clinic-recorded AD patients who had forgotten their past eczema at a rate of approximately 40%; only 70% of the parents remembered the past occurrence in their children. Are there really cases of adult-onset AD in nontropical climates or are they resultant from patient/parent recall failure? Similar to the Naleway study, Moberg and colleagues[12] found that a third of patients with documented AD in childhood had forgotten it by the second or third decade. In their study they confirmed that patients who were more severe and had AD later in life were much more likely to recall that illness. They were also more likely to have hand eczema. That chronic, often recalcitrant, localized problem was seen as 1 factor facilitating the recollection of eczema.

This entire subject is fraught with many crucial points of contrast and conflicting yet poorly documented opinions. Hand eczema is often a late comorbidity associated with AD and it is a frequent one. In the authors' Oregon Health & Science University registry, when 950 AD patients were assessed from 1980 to 1998, 59% had current hand eczema,[13] a figure in line with other studies.[14,15] Many such patients may have only 1

to 2 mild, dorsal hand lesions, which are assumed to be AD combined with contact irritancy and are easily controlled with TCS. Therein lies a possible confusing conflict with dermatologists who insist that large proportions of such patients may actually have allergic contract dermatitis (ACD), with AD considered a lesser possibility. Even with patch testing, the causative distinction between the AD versus ACD is often unclear because patients with AD typically have epidermal barrier defects that can predispose to contact sensitization without actual delayed hypersensitivity lesions. Thus, although all 59% of the authors' hand eczema patients also had AD, and although most were adults, only a small proportion had patch testing and documented ACD. Proof of ACD did not negate the presence of AD based on well-documented criteria.[2] Some studies may also be unreliable because, especially in patients with palmar dominance, psoriasis may have been an underlying predisposition. Psoriasis and eczema are frequently misdiagnosed and patient recall may simply pick one or the other from memory or from family conditions (differential diagnosis of AD presented in **Box 2**). It seems to be useful to obtain biopsies when there is morphologic uncertainty between eczema versus psoriasis. Unfortunately, the biopsy may add uncertainty because many dermatopathologists frequently use the confusing "psoriasiform dermatitis" hedge. The most important indication for biopsy in patients with adult AD is to rule out possible cutaneous T-cell lymphoma.

The bottom line is that whether these cases are adult onset or adult recurrence of AD, they should be diagnosed and managed appropriately as AD.

Management of Atopic Dermatitis in Adults

Physicians experienced in dealing with adult AD tend to agree that management is often difficult. Most experts voice the opinion that childhood AD is much easier to deal with; this may partly reflect skin inflammation levels that are much closer to the surface and within range of safe

> **Box 2**
> **Differential diagnosis in adult atopic dermatitis**
>
> - Allergic contact dermatitis
> - Irritant contact dermatitis
> - Psoriasis
> - Seborrheic dermatitis
> - Cutaneous lymphoma
> - Scabies

TCS control. In adults, the presence of more lichenified lesions creates a higher threshold for the efficacy of topical agents. Plus, the frequency of hand eczema is much greater. Hand eczema remains among the most difficult inflammatory skin problems facing caregivers. If ACD can be proved, then avoidance may be curative, but, for most of these patients, only partial control with medications is possible (**Box 3**).

The lichenification in adult AD, along with the frequent involvement of thick-skinned areas like hands, wrists, ankles, and feet often puts therapeutic responsiveness beyond reach of topical agents. Use of superpotent TCSs is more frequent, yet these often do not provide much relief in areas where the skin is thicker. To help overcome this deficiency, patients are usually advised to practice effective prehydration, such as soaks, swims, or wet cloth coverings, for 20 minutes prior to TCS application.[16] Occlusion with vinyl or nitrile gloves is also used, although, for patients with AD, occlusion can stimulate sweating and the consequent itch can negate the benefit. Perhaps the biggest problem is that optimal compliance with all of these measures occurs at a very low rate.

Prevention and protection are equally important. If hand eczema is unresponsive to recommended hydrations and TCS therapy, patients may need to optimize protection from frequent hand washing and inflammatory stimuli. An ideal approach is to apply white cotton gloves when awakening and cover these with loose-fitting plastic gloves whenever wetting or irritant exposure is encountered. For such patients, patch testing must also

be a strong consideration. Unfortunately, even when a causative allergen is proved, avoidance may be difficult. Deleterious occupational exposures can constitute a situation in which job change could be curative but financial factors make it impossible. Effective protection becomes a less-than-ideal goal.

When all of these efforts fail and the adult eczema persists, consideration must be given to systemic therapies. It probably is best if physicians took an oath to never use systemic corticosteroids beyond a 1-week trial, which, if nonbeneficial, should indicate the much safer and effective approach of prescribing oral cyclosporine A (CsA), even if the recalcitrance only affects the hands. A 2-week trial is indicated and a dose of 5 mg/kg is crucial for quickly assessing benefit in such a recalcitrant problem. Patients generally note onset of pruritic relief within 4 days to 7 days and by 1 month, dosage can begin to taper. Projected duration of (CsA) therapy is usually 6 months to 12 months because lichenification reduces only slowly. When well-controlled, patients can be transitioned to topical agents, to ultraviolet therapy or to other oral agents, such as methotrexate or azathioprine, while CsA is reduced and discontinued. The evolving development of new systemic agents for AD, such as the interleukin 4Rα blocker, dupilumab, and JAK inhibitors, may also bring more effective therapy for those unfortunate patients with adult AD.

In conclusion, adult-onset AD is unable to be classified as a distinct, defined phenotype but more likely as an eczema affecting those Moberg and colleagues[12] labeled "forgetful" patients and parents. This must not distract from the importance of adult AD as an often recalcitrant problem that can be difficult for physicians to manage. It also represents a prominent segment of occupational dermatitis which, in turn, is the largest component of occupational diseases. Involvement limited to the hands causes dermatologists to hesitate with necessary systemic therapy to liberate patients from continuing misery.

Box 3
Factors for assessing atopic dermatitis in adults

- Verify diagnosis: AD versus ACD versus psoriasis
- Personal history of allergies or childhood eczema?—

  "Facial/flexural itch"?

  Ask parents if any childhood "eczema/allergies"?

  Any pediatrician-diagnosed "food allergy"?

- Family history of eczema/allergies
- Occupation—contact with irritants or known contact allergens
- Childhood residence—tropical climate, developing world, or in southern United States or Europe

REFERENCES

1. Hanifin JM, Lobitz WC. Newer concepts of atopic dermatitis. Arch Dermatol 1977;113(5):663–70.
2. Hanifin JM, Rajka G. Diagnostic features of atopic dermatitis. Acta Derm Venereol Suppl 1980;92:44–7.
3. Eichenfield LF, Hanifin JM, Luger TA, et al. Consensus Conference on Pediatric Atopic Dermatitis. J Am Acad Dermatol 2003;49(6):1088–95.
4. Bannister MJ, Freeman S. Adult-onset atopic dermatitis. Australas J Dermatol 2000;41:225–8.

5. Ingordo V, D'Andria G, D'Andria C. Adult-onset atopic dermatitis in a patch test population. Dermatology 2003;206:197–203.

6. Pesce G, Marcon A, Carosso A, et al. Adult eczema in Italy: prevalence and associations with environmental factors. J Eur Acad Dermatol Venereol 2015;29(6):1180–7.

7. Ozkaya E. Adult-onset dermatitis. J Am Acad Dermatol 2005;52:579–82.

8. Katsarou A, Armenaka M. Atopic dermatitis in older patients: particular points. J Eur Acad Dermatol Venereol 2011;25(1):12–8.

9. Lee CH, Chuang HY, Hong CH, et al. Lifetime exposure to cigarette smoking and the development of adult-onset atopic dermatitis. Br J Dermatol 2011; 164:483–9.

10. Thappa DM, Malathi M. Is there something called adult onset atopic dermatitis in India? Indian J Dermatol Venereol Leprol 2013;79:145–7.

11. Naleway AL, Belongia EA, Greenlee RT, et al. Eczematous skin disease and recall of past diagnoses: implications for smallpox vaccination. Ann Intern Med 2003;139:1–7.

12. Moberg C, Meding B, Stenberg B, et al. Remembering childhood atopic dermatitis as an adult: factors that influence recollection. Br J Dermatol 2006; 155:557–60.

13. Simpson EL, Thompson MM, Hanifin JM. Prevalence and morphology of hand eczema in patients with atopic dermatitis. Dermatitis 2006;17(3):123–7.

14. Rystedt I. Work-related hand eczema in atopics. Contact Derm 1985;12:164–71.

15. Meding B. Prevention of hand eczema in atopics. Curr Probl Dermatol 1996;25:116–22.

16. Hajar T, Hanifin JM, Tofte SJ, et al. Prehydration is effective for rapid control of recalcitrant atopic dermatitis. Dermatitis 2014;25(2):56–9.

Patient Burden of Atopic Dermatitis

Cathryn Sibbald, MD[a,b], Aaron M. Drucker, MD[c],*

KEYWORDS

- Eczema • Atopic dermatitis • Burden • Quality of life • Atopy • Itch • Sleep • Outcome measures

KEY POINTS

- Patient burden in atopic dermatitis (AD) is significant and is comparable to other dermatoses without systemic involvement.
- Itch and pain are the most common symptoms in AD, and can have pronounced detrimental effects on quality of life (QoL) and sleep in patients with AD.
- Disease impacts include work and leisure limitations, difficulties in interpersonal relationships, and time lost to management of the disease.
- Most studies demonstrate a significant association between increasing disease severity and worsening impact on QoL.
- Both pharmacologic and educational interventions that improve disease severity appear to simultaneously improve QoL.

INTRODUCTION

Patients with atopic dermatitis (AD) experience symptoms and changes in skin appearance that can have significant impacts on physical and psychosocial health. The resulting negative effects on quality of life (QoL), relationships, and work or school performance can be overwhelming.

Although most cases will resolve before adulthood, AD is often persistent into and can begin in adulthood, resulting in a lifetime patient burden that is one of the largest among diseases worldwide.[1,2] In the 2010 Global Burden of Disease report, 267 diseases were assessed using years lived with disability (YLD). This summary measure is calculated using the prevalence of disease-associated health sequelae multiplied by disability weights to incorporate the extent and duration of the impacts of a disease. Eczema had the 25th highest YLD of all diseases, and the highest among all skin diseases (note: we use the less-specific term "eczema" here, as that is what is used in the primary sources).[3,4]

To address the significant patient burden of AD, clinicians need to understand the main contributors to impaired QoL, possible predictors of more severe impacts, and the effects of different interventions.

MEASUREMENT OF PATIENT BURDEN IN ATOPIC DERMATITIS

Assessment of QoL is important in the management of AD as well as in clinical trials. Although QoL generally correlates with disease severity, they are not always closely related.[5] This suggests that severity as assessed by clinicians does not fully capture the impact on patients. Therefore,

---

Disclosure Statement: Dr A.M. Drucker is an investigator for Sanofi and Regeneron and has received honoraria from Astellas Canada.
[a] Division of Dermatology, University of Toronto, 2075 Bayview Avenue M1-700, Toronto, Ontario M4N 3M5, Canada; [b] Division of Dermatology, Sunnybrook Health Sciences Centre, 2075 Bayview Avenue M1-700, Toronto, Ontario M4N 3M5, Canada; [c] Department of Dermatology, Warren Alpert Medical School, Brown University, Box G-D, Providence, RI 02912, USA
* Corresponding author.
E-mail address: aaron_drucker@brown.edu

Dermatol Clin 35 (2017) 303–316
http://dx.doi.org/10.1016/j.det.2017.02.004
0733-8635/17/© 2017 Elsevier Inc. All rights reserved.

when making therapeutic decisions, clinicians should take the QoL impact of a patient's AD into account and not only rely on assessments of symptoms and signs. For example, a patient with mild disease based on physical examination may have significant impacts on QoL, necessitating more aggressive therapy than their clinical signs would suggest. QoL can be assessed informally with open-ended questions or questions targeting domains known to be affected by AD, such as those detailed in this review. It may be preferable, though, to include a formal assessment of QoL or patient burden in clinical encounters.

A variety of different measures have been used to assess QoL in patients with AD, including generic health, dermatology-specific, and AD-specific scales (Table 1). These scales vary widely in target populations, domains assessed, and scoring algorithms. A recent systematic review of instruments used in AD trials identified 28 different QoL scales used in 45 trials.[6] The heterogeneity of these tools makes it challenging to compare or pool findings of impaired QoL or treatment effects on QoL across different studies. The most commonly used scales include the Dermatology Life Quality Index (DLQI) and the Childhood DLQI (CDLQI), used in more than 40 studies of patients with AD.[7,8] These scales include only 10 items, but cover a large breadth of variables, including symptoms and feelings, daily activities, leisure, work and school, personal relationships, and treatment. Although they target patients with skin disease, a concern is the lack of specificity for AD. An alternative patient-reported outcome measure is the 7-item Patient Oriented Eczema Measure (POEM), which is specific for signs and symptoms of AD, but does not assess impact on activities or psychosocial well-being.[9] Taking only a few minutes to complete, this is an attractive standardized option for assessing and monitoring symptoms in clinical practice.

PREVALENCE OF SYMPTOMS AND IMPAIRED QUALITY OF LIFE IN PATIENTS WITH ATOPIC DERMATITIS
Itch and Pain

Itch perpetuates the dermatitis cycle and is a major component of the diagnostic criteria for AD.[10] In an electronic questionnaire-based study of 304 patients with AD, 91% reported daily itch and 68% experienced itch more than 4 times each day.[11] Most patients who experience itch find it difficult to live with. The National Family Opinion survey in 2001 included 559 respondents with a self-reported history of AD symptoms or diagnosis.[12] In this population, 63.2% of respondents rated their itching (if present) as "very

bothersome" or "extremely bothersome" in the past 12 months.[12] In a pediatric cohort of 120 girls with AD, 95% were troubled by itching and scratching on the DLQI Questionnaire.[13]

The impact of itch on QoL can be pronounced. In addition to correlations between itch and measures of QoL, itch has been correlated with psychological distress, fatigue, and feelings of helplessness.[14] One of the most commonly reported consequences of itch is sleep disturbance.[15–19] In a multicenter cross-sectional survey of 151 children and 172 adults with AD, 87.1% had difficulty falling asleep either frequently or nearly always, and 73.5% stated that itching frequently or nearly always woke them up from sleep.[18]

Many patients with AD experience both pain and itch, and they can be difficult to separate. Some patients may perceive itch as painful, especially as itch intensity increases.[11] In a survey of 1111 patients with AD and parents from 34 countries, more than 80% identified pain/soreness as being "quite important" or "very important" when asked about what factors influence their decision about what treatments are working.[20]

Self-Esteem

Patients with AD may feel self-conscious or embarrassed about the appearance of their skin, with resulting fear and avoidance of going out in public. Classmates or coworkers who tease or bully patients may reinforce these fears.

A study of 336 university students in California explored self-perceived stigma due to skin diseases with an online survey.[21] In 55 participants with a history of eczema, 21.8% reported being bullied or teased, 29.1% perceived being stared at by others, 21.8% had difficulty finding a romantic partner, and 25.5% reported that their eczema affected their social life. The strongest indicator of experiencing stigma was a feeling of awkwardness at being touched or seen by other people, reported in more than half of patients with eczema (58.2%). Fortunately, only a small percentage (3.6%) perceived discrimination at work or school.

In a telephone survey of 2002 patients and caregivers in 8 countries, 27% of adults reported a history of bullying; in children aged 8 to 17 it was even more prevalent at 39%.[22] In the same population, 44% of adults were embarrassed about their appearance, and 53% were concerned about being seen in public.[22]

Sleep Disturbance

Patients with AD may experience a variety of negative effects on sleep, including difficulty falling

Table 1
Comparison of quality of life scales used in studies evaluating patient burden in atopic dermatitis

Scale	Target Age	Length of Survey	Variables/Domains Assessed
General health scales			
SF-36[55]	Adults	36 items (10 min)	Physical functioning (10 items) Limitations due to physical health or emotional problems (7 items) Energy/fatigue (4 items) Emotional well-being (5 items) Social functioning (2 items) Pain (2 items) General health (5 items)
SF-12[56]	Adults (age >18 y)	12 items (2–3 min)	Physical functioning (2 items) Limitations due to physical health or emotional problems (4 items) Energy/fatigue (1 item) Emotional well-being (1 item) Social functioning (1 item) Pain (1 item) General health (2 items)
EQ-5D[57]	Adults	6 items (5 min)	1 item for each of 5 domains: Mobility, self-care, usual activities, pain/discomfort, anxiety/depression + Visual Analogue Scale rating quality of overall health
Dermatology-specific scales			
DLQI[8]	Adults	10 items (2 min)	Symptoms and feelings (2 items) Daily activities (2 items) Leisure (2 items) Work and school (1 item) Personal relationships (2 items) Treatment (1 item)
CDLQI[58]	Children 3–16 y old	10 items (2 min)	Same as DLQI
Skindex-29[59]	Adults	30 items (5 min)	Symptoms (7 items) Emotions (10 items) Functioning (12 items)
Atopic dermatitis–specific scales			
IDQOL[60]	Parents of infants younger than 4 y	10 items (2–3 min)	Symptoms and mood (2 items) Sleep (2 items) Leisure (2 items) Daily activities (3 item) Treatment (1 item)
CADIS[61]	Children <6 y and their parents	45 items (6 min)	Child symptoms (7 items) Child activity limitations and behavior (9 items) Family and social function (9 items) Parent sleep (3 items) Parent emotions (17 items)

Abbreviations: CADIS, childhood atopic dermatitis impact scale; CDLQI, Childhood Dermatology Life Quality Index; DLQI, Dermatology Life Quality Index; EQ-5D, European Quality of Life-5 dimensions; IDQOL, Infant's Dermatitis Quality of Life Index; SF-36, Medical Outcomes Short Form-36 Health Survey.

asleep, frequent awakenings, shorter overall duration of sleep, or sleep fragmentation. In 1 study of 148 children with AD and 2937 without, sleep duration was significantly shorter in those with severe dermatitis compared with controls (542 ± 67 vs 569 ± 62 minutes nightly, $P = .02$).[23]

Sleep is often closely linked with pruritus, as patients may experience difficulty falling asleep or frequent awakenings with itch. In a polysomnography and actigraphy study, total scratching index was significantly correlated with percentage of body surface area affected with eczema (0.333, $P = -.008$), polysomnographic sleep efficiency (-0.56, $P = .10$) and Actigraph sleep efficiency (-0.52, $P = .019$).[24] For this study, sleep efficiency was defined by the ratio of total sleep time to time in bed.

Poor sleep may lead to poor overall physical health and increased risk of injury, with supporting evidence from 3 US population-based studies. The first included 34,613 adults and reported that fatigue in patients with AD was associated with an increased risk of self-perceived fair or poor health (odds ratio [OR] 8.63, 95% confidence interval [CI] 7.15–10.43).[25] Pooled data from 9 different population-based studies of 264,326 children reported increased odds of having a height less than the fifth percentile in adolescents aged 10 to 11 years old with AD and 0 to 3 nights of sufficient sleep per week.[26] In a US population-based survey of 2484 patients with AD, adults with AD and fatigue (adjusted OR 2.61, 95% CI 1.91–3.55), daytime sleepiness (2.31, 1.69–3.16), or insomnia (2.62, 1.94–3.55) had higher rates of fractures and bone or joint injuries compared with those without AD.[27]

Impact on Participation in Leisure and Sports

AD also can significantly impact participation in social and sport activities. Patients may feel reluctant to participate because of fear of stigmatization, teasing or bullying, or because of symptoms that worsen with heat or sweating. In a postal survey of 117 children with AD in the Netherlands, 31% to 35% reported avoiding social activities, and 35% to 43% reported avoiding sports activities.[28] In this study, the motivation for avoiding these activities may have been due to feeling shame from peers, which was reported in 64% to 70% of participants.

Impact on Attendance and Performance at School and Work

AD can have direct and indirect effects on work or school performance. In US population-based surveys of 61,770 participants, eczema was associated with more than 50% increased odds of missing more than 5 days of work in each of 2010 (OR 1.59, 95% CI 1.34–1.88) and 2012 (OR 1.53, 95% CI 1.26–1.84).[29] In that study, there was no correlation between severity of eczema and number of days missed, whereas in a smaller Canadian study of 76 patients, 43% with severe disease missed at least 1 day of work compared

with 10% with mild disease and 5% with moderate disease.[30]

Although those studies demonstrate increased time away from work or school among people with AD, there is no convincing evidence of an impact on school performance. In a cross-sectional survey of 3553 adolescents in Norway including 346 patients with AD, there was no significant increase in self-reports of "not thriving in school" despite a higher prevalence of mental health problems.[31] These findings were supported in a birth cohort of 1865 children in the Netherlands, 51% of whom suffered from eczema. Review of teacher assessments of these participants at an age of 17 years did not reveal any association between presence or duration of AD and standardized tests or school performance.[32]

Patients with AD are at higher risk of hand dermatitis, which may be especially impactful on school and work performance, given the need to use one's hands in many activities and occupations. In a case control study of 783 participants, including 405 cases with a history of childhood AD, hand eczema was significantly more common in patients with AD (41.8% vs 13.4%, $P<.01$).[33] In this population, 10% reported taking more than 7 days of sick leave due to eczema. Missed work can have many negative implications, including missed income and concerns of job security.

Impact on Career Choice

In addition to the immediate effects of AD on work productivity, long-term and broad effects are possible, including the avoidance of certain careers or employment opportunities. In a cross-sectional survey of 100 patients in Denmark, 38% reported occupation or job avoidance because of their eczema, including avoiding work in nursing, physiotherapy in pools, surgery, veterinary medicine, catering, cooking, farming, automobile repair, hair dressing, and cleaning.[34] Restriction of such a large range of occupations could not only affect job and career satisfaction, but also prevent societal benefit from potential talented and successful workers.

Patients with AD also may perceive an impact on how they are treated by employers or co-workers, and the opportunities that they are offered. In 1088 adult patients surveyed in a multicenter study, 11% felt discriminated against because of their AD, and 14% believed that their career progression was hindered.[22] More research would be helpful in determining if these impacts are related to disease severity or other patient demographics.

Table 2
Impact of systemic treatment on QoL

Study	Study Design	Setting	Target Population	Sample Size	Average Age, y	Main Outcomes	Interventions	Results
Haeck et al,[62] 2011	Randomized controlled trial	Tertiary center in Germany, Nov 2005–2007	Adults with severe AD	49	37.3 ± 12.9	QoL: DLQI Efficacy: SCORAD, SASSAD	CsA 5 mg/kg × 6 wk then CsA 3 mg/kg OR mycophenolate sodium 1440 mg/d	CsA: improved disease activity (SCORAD, SASSAD, "rule of 9s") of 10 points associated with improvement of 1.3, 1.5, 1.1 points, respectively, in DLQI[5] Mycophenolate: specific results not reported
Salek et al,[63] 1993	Crossover randomized control Trial	Multicenter in the United Kingdom, Dates NS	Adults with severe AD	33	Group A: Median 29 (16–58) Group B: Median 30 (16–43)	QoL: EDI and UKSIP Efficacy: clinical scores	Group A: placebo × 8 wk then CsA 5 mg/kg × 8 wk Group B: CsA 5 mg/kg × 8 wk then placebo × 8 wk	68% (Group A) and 26% (Group B) improvement in UKSIP after CsA: Group A: 5.6 ± 1.8–1.8 ± 1.2 Group B: 6.5 ± 1.7–4.8 ± 1.9 74% (Group A) and 49% (Group B) improvement in EDI after CsA: Group A: 29.1 ± 4.8–7.6 ± 1.7 Group B: 33.2 ± 4.7–16.1 ± 5.3
Berth-Jones et al,[64] 1996	Open-label study	Multicenter, United Kingdom, Dates NS	Children with severe AD	27	9 (2–16)	QoL: 31-item questionnaire Efficacy: Rule of 9s	CsA 5 mg/kg/d × 6 wk	56% improvement in QoL scores at week 6 (n = 24) and 68% at week 8 (n = 18): Mean QoL: 44 at baseline, 24.8 at week 6, 29.7 at week 8 Standard deviations not reported

(continued on next page)

Table 2
(continued)

Study	Study Design	Setting	Target Population	Sample Size	Average Age, y	Main Outcomes	Interventions	Results
Harper et al,[65] 2000	Prospective randomized parallel group study	Multicenter, United Kingdom, June 1995–December 1997	Children with severe AD	40	10 (3–16)	QoL: CDLQI Efficacy: SASSAD	CsA 5 mg/kg/d: either 12 wk then taper or continuous (with possible restart and dose adjustments per protocol)	Improved CDLQI in short course and continuous arm at week 12 ($P = .004$ and $P = .0004$, respectively) Significant difference from baseline at 1 y only in continuous arm ($P = .01$) despite similar efficacy scores, and better QoL scores at week 12 vs year 1 Specific results not reported
Czech et al,[66] 2000	Prospective randomized double-blind parallel group study	21 centers in Germany	Adults with severe AD	106	34 (18–63)	QoL: DLQI Efficacy: TBSA	CsA 150 mg or 300 mg daily × 8 wk	41.4% (150 mg group) and 57.4% (300 mg) improvement in DLQI Scores at 8 wk: 150 mg group: 15 ± 7.3– 8.8 ± 7.4 300 mg group: 15.5 ± 7.5–6.6 ± 6.5 (in parallel with improved TBSA scores)
Lyakhovitsky et al,[67] 2010	Retrospective review	Dermatology outpatient clinic in Israel, Aug 2004–April 2008	Adults with moderate-severe AD	20	51.75 ± 18.27	QoL: DLQI Efficacy: SCORAD	MTX 10–25 mg once weekly × 8–12 wk	16 patients responded 43.5% improvement in DLQI Mean SCORAD + DLQI decreased by 28.65 units (44.3%) and 10.15 units (43.5%) respectively The decrease in DLQI was more significant in the adult-onset than in the childhood-onset group (10.7 ± 7.6 vs 8.4 ± 11.5, respectively)

Study	Study Design	Location	Population	N	Age	Measures	Intervention	Results
Schram et al,[68] 2011	Randomized controlled trial	Amsterdam, the Netherlands, July 2009–December 2010	Adults with severe AD	42	Methotrexate: 43.0 ± 14.7 Azathioprine: 37.0 ± 14.1	QoL: Skindex-17 Efficacy: SCORAD	MTX (10–22.5 mg/wk) × 12 wk (n = 20) Azathioprine (1.5–2.5 mg/kg/d) × 12 wk (n = 22), then 12-wk follow-up	MTX: 25% improvement in QoL Mean Skindex-17 decreased from 50.2 (SD 11.7) to 37.8 (SD 9.8) at week 12 (P<.001) Azathioprine: 19.7% improvement in QoL Mean Skindex-decreased from 51.7 (SD 8.6) to 41.5 (SD 13.1; P<.001).
Panahi et al,[69] 2012	Prospective single-arm study	Tertiary multicenter, Baqiyatallah, Iran	Adults with severe AD	20	38.9 ± 10.96	QoL: DLQI Efficacy: SCORAD	Recombinant human interferon gamma 50 μg/m² SC 3 times a week × 1 mo	60.6% improvement in DLQI: Baseline 20.80 ± 3.95–8.20 ± 2.14 after treatment (P<.001) DLQI score improvement correlated significantly with improved SCORAD
Samrao et al,[70] 2012	Prospective open-label randomized trial	Tertiary center, Oregon	Adults with moderate to severe AD	16	Group A: median age 38 Group B: median age 45	QoL: DLQI Efficacy: EASI	Group A: Apremilast 20 mg PO BID × 3 mo Group B: Apremilast 30 mg PO BID × 6 mo	63.4% (Group A) and 62% (Group B) improvement in DLQI at 3 mo: Group A: mean 14.2–6.2, P<.05 Group B: mean 10.1–3.8, P<.05 Group B: sustained average score of 4.1 at 6 mo, P<.05 Improved DLQI correlated with significant decreases in the EASI score

(continued on next page)

Table 2
(continued)

Study	Study Design	Setting	Target Population	Sample Size	Average Age, y	Main Outcomes	Interventions	Results
Thaçi et al,[51] 2015; Simpson et al,[52] 2016	Randomized placebo-controlled trial	International multicenter trial	Adults with moderate to severe AD	379	Group 1: 36.2 ± 10.7 Group 2: 39.4 ± 12.1 Group 3: 35.8 ± 14.9 Group 4: 36.8 ± 10.8 Group 5: 36.6 ± 11.6 Group 6: 37.2 ± 13.1	QoL: DLQI Efficacy: EASI, SCORAD, TBSA, pruritus scores	Group 1: Dupilumab 300 mg once weekly Group 2: Dupilumab 300 mg every 2 wk Group 3: Dupilumab 200 mg every 2 wk Group 4: Dupilumab 300 mg every 4 wk Group 5: Dupilumab 100 mg every 4 wk Group 6: placebo once weekly	Improvement in DLQI at 16 wk: 71.3% (Group 1), 54.5% (Group 2), 52.7% (Group 3), 48.9% (Group 4), 24.2% (Group 5), 10.2% (Group 6). DLQI scores from baseline to week 16: Group 1: 15.0 ± 7.80–4.3 ± 4.88, $P<.0001$ Group 2: 14·5 ± 7·20–6.6 ± 6.77, $P<.0001$ Group 3: 15.0 ± 7.07–7.1 ± 7.61, $P<.0001$ Group 4: 13.3 ± 7.29–6.8 ± 6.85, $P<.0001$ Group 5: 15.7 ± 6.61–11.9 ± 8.28, $P = .12$ Group 6: 12.8 ± 6.20–11.4 ± 7.18, NS Improved DLQI correlated with significant decreases in the EASI + SCORAD scores

Simpson et al,[50] 2016	2 Randomized double-blind, placebo-controlled trials (SOLO1 and SOLO2)	International multicenter trial	Adults with moderate to severe AD	SOLO1: 671 SOLO2: 708	Median age (IQR)	QoL: DLQI Efficacy: EASI, SCORAD, TBSA, pruritus scores	Both SOLO1 + 2:	Improvement in DLQI at 16 wk:
					SOLO1:		Group 1: placebo once weekly	SOLO1: 37.9% (Group 1, placebo), 71.5% (Group 2), 64.3% (Group 3)
					Group 1: 39.0 (27.0–50.5)		Group 2: Dupilumab 300 mg once weekly	SOLO2: 24% (Group 1, placebo), 62% (Group 2), 59.4% (Group 3)
					Group 2: 38.0 (27.5–48.0)		Group 3: Dupilumab 300 mg every 2 wk	Median baseline DLQI (IQR) and average least mean squares change ($\pm$SD) at wk 16:
					Group 3: 39.0 (27.0–51.0)			SOLO1:
					SOLO2:			Placebo: 14.0 (9.0–20.0), -5.3 ± 0.5
					Group 1: 35.0 (25.0–47.0)			Group 2: 13.0 (8.0–19.0), -9.3 ± 0.4, $P<.001$
					Group 2: 34.0 (25.0–46.0)			Group 3: 14.0 (8.0–20.0), -9.0 ± 0.4, $P<.001$
					Group 3: 35.0 (25.0–46.0)			SOLO2:
								Placebo: 15.0 (9.0–22.0), -3.6 ± 0.5
								Group 2: 15.0 (10.0–21.0), -9.3 ± 0.4, $P<.001$
								Group 3: 16.0 (10.0–22.0), -9.5 ± 0.4, $P<.001$
								Improved DLQI correlated with significant decreases in the EASI + SCORAD scores

(continued on next page)

Table 2
(continued)

Study	Study Design	Setting	Target Population	Sample Size	Average Age, y	Main Outcomes	Interventions	Results
Simpson et al,[49] 2016	2 randomized double-blind, vehicle-controlled trials	Multicenter within the United States	Children and adults with mild to moderate AD affecting >5% BSA	1522	Crisaborole: 12.3 (2–79) Vehicle: 12.1 (2–79)	QoL: CDLQI, DLQI Efficacy: ISGA	Crisaborole 2% ung BID × 28 d Vehicle BID × 28 d	49.5% improvement in CDLQI (P<.001) and 54% improvement in DLQI (P = .016) at Day 29: Mean CDLQI at baseline and day 29: Crisaborole: 9.3 (5.99) to 4.7 Vehicle: 9.0 (6.02) to 6.0 Mean DLQI at baseline and day 29: Crisaborole: 9.7 (6.29) to 4.5 Vehicle: 9.3 (6.55) to 5.8 Improved CDLQI + DLQI correlated with improved ISGA scores

Abbreviations: AD, atopic dermatitis; BID, twice a day; BSA, body surface area; CsA, cyclosporine; EASI, eczema area severity index; EDI, eczema area severity index; ISGA, Investigator's Static Global Assessment; MTX, methotrexate; NS, not specified; PO, by mouth; QoL, quality of life; SASSAD, six area, Six Sign Atopic Dermatitis Severity Score; SC, subcutaneous; SCORAD, Severity Scoring of Atopic Dermatitis; TBSA, total body surface area; UKSIP, United Kingdom sickness impact profile.

Impact on Relationships

AD has been demonstrated to have detrimental effects at home, impacting relationships with both family members and partners. A survey of 6518 adolescents aged 11 to 17 from 2003 to 2006 included 295 patients with AD, using KINDL-R(evised), which measures QoL in the past 7 days over 6 dimensions.[35] In those with eczema, there was a significantly lower self-reported quality of relationships with family compared with adolescents without AD, with KINDL-R scores of 79.08 ± 0.91 compared with 82.12 ± 0.21 out of 100, P = .002. In another cross-sectional study of 1098 adults with AD, 21% found it difficult to form relationships with their partners because of their disease.[22]

Time Spent Managing Atopic Dermatitis

Patients with AD and their families often devote a lot of time to their illness. Activities include medical appointments, possible emergency visits or hospital admissions, filling prescriptions, and applying topical treatments. In a study of 42 children with AD in Denmark in 2001, the total average time spent on treatment was estimated to be 62 minutes daily.[36] Not only are these activities burdensome, but the time devoted to them is lost from other potential work or pleasure activities.

EFFECTS OF TREATMENT ON QUALITY OF LIFE IN PATIENTS WITH ATOPIC DERMATITIS

Many AD treatment studies include QoL measures, and almost all report improvement of QoL measures that parallel response to treatment.

Several large studies have evaluated the impact of topical calcineurin inhibitors on QoL. According to these studies, treatment with topical tacrolimus and pimecrolimus improves QoL in parallel with improvements in disease severity in children and adults.[37-48] One of the largest of these was a postmarketing surveillance study of patients with AD using pimecrolimus cream in 5665 participants.[46] After 6 weeks of treatment, there was a 6-point average decrease in DLQI score in 1773 adults, and a 7.5-point average decrease in CDLQI score in 1438 children. These changes coincided with marked reduction in AD symptoms.

Similarly, the new topical PDE4 inhibitor, crisaborole, demonstrated improved CDLQI and DLQI scores in 797 children and 192 adults with mild to moderate disease by 47.5% and 54.0%, respectively, after only 4 weeks of twice-daily application of the 2% ointment.[49] These changes were significantly better than patients randomized to vehicle, and correlated with improved severity

scores. Trials of longer duration with active comparators are needed to define the full benefit of crisaborole.

Many trials evaluating the impact of systemic therapies on QoL have reported improvements in QoL that paralleled improvement in disease severity indices (**Table 2**). These data are limited by mostly small sample sizes, heterogeneous outcome measures, and patient demographics. One of the largest studies reported the effect of 6 weeks of cyclosporine on DLQI in 54 patients.[5] Interestingly, significant improvements in disease severity as measured by the SCORAD (Severity Scoring of Atopic Dermatitis) were associated with only very minor improvements in DLQI scores, which did not reach statistical significance.

More recently, larger trials have evaluated QoL impacts of the monoclonal antibody dupilumab.[50-52] In phase 2 and 3 trials of 379 and 1379 patients, respectively, DLQI scores improved after 16 weeks of therapy in a dose-dependent manner, with 51% to 72% improvement in DLQI at doses of 300 mg every 1 or 2 weeks.

A different approach to improving QoL in patients with AD involves educational interventions, with 2 studies to date. The first study evaluated a Web site intervention in 143 caregivers of children with AD, and reported benefits in POEM scores from the Web site group.[53] Unfortunately, although QoL measures were collected, these were not reported in this study. The other study randomized 992 parents of children with AD to weekly group education sessions for 6 weeks, and reported significant improvements in QoL and disease severity in the intervention groups.[54] These results highlight the importance and key integral role of education and patient support in care, and suggest possible benefits for QoL.

SUMMARY

AD creates a significant burden on patients. Knowledge of the key contributors to decreased QoL can direct clinicians to better assess burden on an individual basis. Validated tools to assess QoL can be helpful in assessing or monitoring patient burden and response to treatment, and can be incorporated relatively easily into routine clinical care, especially those that can be answered and scored quickly and simply at a patient's appointment.[8,9] In lieu of these standardized tools, clinicians also may focus on patient burden in their general histories, including assessments of symptoms of itch and pain, sleep disturbance, time spent on care, work and leisure limitations, and any negative psychological symptoms. A QoL impact that is divergent from what is expected based on physical examination could provide impetus for more or less aggressive treatment strategies, and can be used to help define treatment goals and assess effectiveness.

Both pharmacologic and educational interventions that improve disease severity appear to simultaneously improve QoL, but some components may be easier influenced in milder or less chronic disease. Hopefully, more research in this area will help identify the most effective interventions, and help clarify if subpopulations can be specifically targeted to improve QoL and patient burden.

REFERENCES

1. Hanifin JM, Reed ML, Eczema Prevalence and Impact Working Group. A population-based survey of eczema prevalence in the United States. Dermatitis 2007;18(2):82–91.
2. Kim JP, Chao LX, Simpson EL, et al. Persistence of atopic dermatitis (AD): a systematic review and meta-analysis. J Am Acad Dermatol 2016;75(4): 681–7.e11.
3. Hay RJ, Johns NE, Williams HC, et al. The global burden of skin disease in 2010: an analysis of the prevalence and impact of skin conditions. J Invest Dermatol 2014;134(6):1527–34.
4. Murray CJ, Atkinson C, Bhalla K, et al. The state of US health, 1990-2010: burden of diseases, injuries, and risk factors. JAMA 2013;310(6):591–608.
5. Haeck IM, ten Berge O, van Velsen SG, et al. Moderate correlation between quality of life and disease activity in adult patients with atopic dermatitis. J Eur Acad Dermatol Venereol 2012;26(2):236–41.
6. Hill MK, Kheirandish Pishkenari A, Braunberger TL, et al. Recent trends in disease severity and quality of life instruments for patients with atopic dermatitis: a systematic review. J Am Acad Dermatol 2016; 75(5):906–17.
7. Beattie PE, Lewis-Jones MS. A comparative study of impairment of quality of life in children with skin disease and children with other chronic childhood diseases. Br J Dermatol 2006;155(1):145–51.
8. Finlay AY, Khan GK. Dermatology Life Quality Index (DLQI)–a simple practical measure for routine clinical use. Clin Exp Dermatol 1994;19(3):210–6.
9. Charman CR, Venn AJ, Williams HC, et al. The patient-oriented eczema measure: development and initial validation of a new tool for measuring atopic eczema severity from the patients' perspective. Arch Dermatol 2004;140(12):1513–9.
10. Williams HC, Burney PG, Pembroke AC, et al. The U.K. Working Party's Diagnostic Criteria for Atopic Dermatitis. III. Independent hospital validation. Br J Dermatol 1994;131(3):406–16.
11. Dawn A, Papoiu AD, Chan YH, et al. Itch characteristics in atopic dermatitis: results of a web-based questionnaire. Br J Dermatol 2009;160(3):642–4.
12. Anderson RT, Rajagopalan R. Effects of allergic dermatosis on health-related quality of life. Curr Allergy Asthma Rep 2001;1(4):309–15.
13. Ballardini N, Ostblom E, Wahlgren CF, et al. Mild eczema affects self-perceived health among pre-adolescent girls. Acta Derm Venereol 2014;94(3): 312–6.
14. Evers AW, Lu Y, Duller P, et al. Common burden of chronic skin diseases? Contributors to psychological distress in adults with psoriasis and atopic dermatitis. Br J Dermatol 2005;152(6):1275–81.
15. Chrostowska-Plak D, Reich A, Szepietowski JC, et al. Relationship between itch and psychological status of patients with atopic dermatitis. J Eur Acad Dermatol Venereol 2013;27(2):e239–242.
16. Langenbruch A, Radtke M, Franzke N, et al. Quality of health care of atopic eczema in Germany: results of the national health care study AtopicHealth. J Eur Acad Dermatol Venereol 2014;28(6):719–26.
17. LeBovidge JS, Kelley SD, Lauretti A, et al. Integrating medical and psychological health care for children with atopic dermatitis. J Pediatr Psychol 2007;32(5):617–25.
18. Sanchez-Perez J, Dauden-Tello E, Mora AM, et al. Impact of atopic dermatitis on health-related quality of life in Spanish children and adults: the PSEDA study. Actas Dermosifiliogr 2013;104(1):44–52.
19. Yosipovitch G, Goon AT, Wee J, et al. Itch characteristics in Chinese patients with atopic dermatitis using a new questionnaire for the assessment of pruritus. Int J Dermatol 2002;41(4):212–6.
20. von Kobyletzki LB, Thomas KS, Schmitt J, et al. What factors are important to patients when assessing treatment response: an international cross-sectional survey. Acta Derm Venereol 2017;96(7): 86–90.
21. Roosta N, Black DS, Peng D, et al. Skin disease and stigma in emerging adulthood: impact on healthy development. J Cutan Med Surg 2010;14(6):285–90.
22. Zuberbier T, Orlow SJ, Paller AS, et al. Patient perspectives on the management of atopic dermatitis. J Allergy Clin Immunol 2006;118(1):226–32.
23. Anuntaseree W, Sangsupawanich P, Osmond C, et al. Sleep quality in infants with atopic dermatitis: a community-based, birth cohort study. Asian Pac J Allergy Immunol 2012;30(1):26–31.
24. Bender BG, Ballard R, Canono B, et al. Disease severity, scratching, and sleep quality in patients with atopic dermatitis. J Am Acad Dermatol 2008; 58(3):415–20.
25. Silverberg JI, Garg NK, Paller AS, et al. Sleep disturbances in adults with eczema are associated with impaired overall health: a US population-based study. J Invest Dermatol 2015;135(1):56–66.

26. Silverberg JI, Paller AS. Association between eczema and stature in 9 US population-based studies. JAMA Dermatol 2015;151(4):401–9.

27. Garg N, Silverberg JI. Association between eczema and increased fracture and bone or joint injury in adults: a US population-based study. JAMA Dermatol 2015;151(1):33–41.

28. Brenninkmeijer EE, Legierse CM, Sillevis Smitt JH, et al. The course of life of patients with childhood atopic dermatitis. Pediatr Dermatol 2009;26(1):14–22.

29. Silverberg JI. Health care utilization, patient costs, and access to care in US adults with eczema: a population-based study. JAMA Dermatol 2015; 151(7):743–52.

30. Barbeau M, Bpharm HL. Burden of atopic dermatitis in Canada. Int J Dermatol 2006;45(1):31–6.

31. Halvorsen JA, Lien L, Dalgard F, et al. Suicidal ideation, mental health problems, and social function in adolescents with eczema: a population-based study. J Invest Dermatol 2014;134(7):1847–54.

32. Ruijsbroek A, Wijga AH, Gehring U, et al. School performance: a matter of health or socio-economic background? Findings from the PIAMA Birth Cohort Study. PLoS One 2015;10(8):e0134780.

33. Nyren M, Lindberg M, Stenberg B, et al. Influence of childhood atopic dermatitis on future worklife. Scand J Work Environ Health 2005;31(6):474–8.

34. Holm EA, Esmann S, Jemec GB. The handicap caused by atopic dermatitis–sick leave and job avoidance. J Eur Acad Dermatol Venereol 2006; 20(3):255–9.

35. Matterne U, Schmitt J, Diepgen TL, et al. Children and adolescents' health-related quality of life in relation to eczema, asthma and hay fever: results from a population-based cross-sectional study. Qual Life Res 2011;20(8):1295–305.

36. Holm EA, Jemec GB. Time spent on treatment of atopic dermatitis: a new method of measuring pediatric morbidity? Pediatr Dermatol 2004;21(6):623–7.

37. De Backer M, Morren MA, Boonen H, et al. Belgian observational drug utilization study of pimecrolimus cream 1% in routine daily practice in atopic dermatitis. Dermatology 2008;217(2):156–63.

38. Drake L, Prendergast M, Maher R, et al. The impact of tacrolimus ointment on health-related quality of life of adult and pediatric patients with atopic dermatitis. J Am Acad Dermatol 2001;44(1 Suppl):S65–72.

39. Kawashima M. QOL research forum for patients with atopic dermatitis. quality of life in patients with atopic dermatitis: impact of tacrolimus ointment. Int J Dermatol 2006;45(6):731–6.

40. Kim KH, Kono T. Overview of efficacy and safety of tacrolimus ointment in patients with atopic dermatitis in Asia and other areas. Int J Dermatol 2011;50(9): 1153–61.

41. Kondo Y, Nakajima Y. QOL research forum for patients with atopic dermatitis. Short-term efficacy of tacrolimus ointment and impact on quality of life. Pediatr Int 2009;51(3):385–9.

42. Poole CD, Chambers C, Sidhu MK, et al. Health-related utility among adults with atopic dermatitis treated with 0.1% tacrolimus ointment as maintenance therapy over the long term: findings from the Protopic CONTROL study. Br J Dermatol 2009; 161(6):1335–40.

43. Reitamo S, Ortonne JP, Sand C, et al. Long-term treatment with 0.1% tacrolimus ointment in adults with atopic dermatitis: results of a two-year, multicentre, non-comparative study. Acta Derm Venereol 2007;87(5):406–12.

44. Singalavanija S, Noppakun N, Limpongsanuruk W, et al. Efficacy and safety of tacrolimus ointment in pediatric patients with moderate to severe atopic dermatitis. J Med Assoc Thai 2006;89(11): 1915–22.

45. Staab D, Kaufmann R, Bräutigam M, et al. Treatment of infants with atopic eczema with pimecrolimus cream 1% improves parents' quality of life: a multicenter, randomized trial. Pediatr Allergy Immunol 2005;16(6):527–33.

46. Sunderkotter C, Weiss JM, Bextermöller R, et al. Post-marketing surveillance on treatment of 5,665 patients with atopic dermatitis using the calcineurin inhibitor pimecrolimus: positive effects on major symptoms of atopic dermatitis and on quality of life. J Dtsch Dermatol Ges 2006;4(4):301–6 [in German].

47. Whalley D, Huels J, McKenna SP, et al. The benefit of pimecrolimus (Elidel, SDZ ASM 981) on parents' quality of life in the treatment of pediatric atopic dermatitis. Pediatrics 2002;110(6):1133–6.

48. Won CH, Seo PG, Park YM, et al. A multicenter trial of the efficacy and safety of 0.03% tacrolimus ointment for atopic dermatitis in Korea. J Dermatolog Treat 2004;15(1):30–4.

49. Simpson E, Paller A, Boguniewicz M, et al. O063 Crisaborole demonstrates improvement in quality of life in patients with mild to moderate atopic dermatitis. Ann Allergy Asthma Immunol 2016;117(Issue Suppl):S20–1.

50. Simpson EL, Bieber T, Guttman-Yassky E, et al. Two phase 3 trials of dupilumab versus placebo in atopic dermatitis. N Engl J Med 2016;75(24):2335–48.

51. Thaci D, Simpson EL, Beck LA, et al. Efficacy and safety of dupilumab in adults with moderate-to-severe atopic dermatitis inadequately controlled by topical treatments: a randomised, placebo-controlled, dose-ranging phase 2b trial. Lancet 2016;387(10013):40–52.

52. Simpson EL, Gadkari A, Worm M, et al. Dupilumab therapy provides clinically meaningful improvement in patient-reported outcomes (PROs): a phase IIb, randomized, placebo-controlled, clinical trial in adult patients with moderate to severe atopic dermatitis (AD). J Am Acad Dermatol 2016;75(3):506–15.

53. Santer M, Muller I, Yardley L, et al. Supporting self-care for families of children with eczema with a Web-based intervention plus health care professional support: pilot randomized controlled trial. J Med Internet Res 2014;16(3):e70.

54. Staab D, Diepgen TL, Fartasch M, et al. Age related, structured educational programmes for the management of atopic dermatitis in children and adolescents: multicentre, randomised controlled trial. BMJ 2006;332(7547):933–8.

55. Brazier JE, Harper R, Jones NM, et al. Validating the SF-36 health survey questionnaire: new outcome measure for primary care. BMJ 1992;305(6846): 160–4.

56. Gandek B, Ware JE, Aaronson NK, et al. Cross-validation of item selection and scoring for the SF-12 Health Survey in nine countries: results from the IQOLA Project. International Quality of Life Assessment. J Clin Epidemiol 1998;51(11):1171–8.

57. Rabin R, de Charro F. EQ-5D: a measure of health status from the EuroQol Group. Ann Med 2001; 33(5):337–43.

58. Lewis-Jones MS, Finlay AY. The Children's Dermatology Life Quality Index (CDLQI): initial validation and practical use. Br J Dermatol 1995;132(6):942–9.

59. Chren MM, Lasek RJ, Flocke SA, et al. Improved discriminative and evaluative capability of a refined version of Skindex, a quality-of-life instrument for patients with skin diseases. Arch Dermatol 1997; 133(11):1433–40.

60. Lewis-Jones MS, Finlay AY, Dykes PJ, et al. The infants' dermatitis quality of life index. Br J Dermatol 2001;144(1):104–10.

61. Chamlin SL, Cella D, Frieden IJ, et al. Development of the Childhood Atopic Dermatitis Impact Scale: initial validation of a quality-of-life measure for young children with atopic dermatitis and their families. J Invest Dermatol 2005;125(6):1106–11.

62. Haeck IM, Knol MJ, Ten Berge O, et al. Enteric-coated mycophenolate sodium versus cyclosporin A as long-term treatment in adult patients with severe atopic dermatitis: a randomized controlled trial. J Am Acad Dermatol 2011;64(6):1074–84.

63. Salek MS, Finlay AY, Luscombe DK, et al. Cyclosporin greatly improves the quality of life of adults with severe atopic dermatitis. A randomized, double-blind, placebo-controlled trial. Br J Dermatol 1993;129(4):422–30.

64. Berth-Jones J, Finlay AY, Zaki I, et al. Cyclosporine in severe childhood atopic dermatitis: a multicenter study. J Am Acad Dermatol 1996;34(6):1016–21.

65. Harper JI, Ahmed I, Barclay G, et al. Cyclosporin for severe childhood atopic dermatitis: short course versus continuous therapy. Br J Dermatol 2000; 142(1):52–8.

66. Czech W, Brautigam M, Weidinger G, et al. A body-weight-independent dosing regimen of cyclosporine microemulsion is effective in severe atopic dermatitis and improves the quality of life. J Am Acad Dermatol 2000;42(4):653–9.

67. Lyakhovitsky A, Barzilai A, Heyman R, et al. Low-dose methotrexate treatment for moderate-to-severe atopic dermatitis in adults. J Eur Acad Dermatol Venereol 2010;24(1):43–9.

68. Schram ME, Roekevisch E, Leeflang MM, et al. A randomized trial of methotrexate versus azathioprine for severe atopic eczema. J Allergy Clin Immunol 2011;128(2):353–9.

69. Panahi Y, Davoudi SM, Madanchi N, et al. Recombinant human interferon gamma (Gamma Immunex) in treatment of atopic dermatitis. Clin Exp Med 2012; 12(4):241–5.

70. Samrao A, Berry TM, Goreshi R, et al. A pilot study of an oral phosphodiesterase inhibitor (apremilast) for atopic dermatitis in adults. Arch Dermatol 2012; 148(8):890–7.

An Update on the Pathophysiology of Atopic Dermatitis

Kunal Malik, BA[a,b,c,1], Kerry D. Heitmiller, BA[d,2],
Tali Czarnowicki, MD, MSc[a,b],*

KEYWORDS

- Atopic dermatitis • Pathophysiology • Epithelial barrier • Immune dysregulation • Microbiome

KEY POINTS

- Atopic dermatitis (AD) is increasingly recognized as multifactorial and heterogeneous with differing molecular or cellular phenotypes characterizing different populations.
- Accumulating studies continue clarifying key interactions among susceptibility genes, environmental factors, microbiome, impaired barrier integrity, and immune dysregulation.
- Identification of immune subsets, including Th17, Th22, and Th9, has shifted disease paradigms from biphasic Th1/Th2 driven to a complex, multi-axes disease.
- Advances in AD pathomechanisms are leading to robust development of novel, targeted therapeutics, whereas current treatments are limited and may harbor toxic effects.

INTRODUCTION

Atopic dermatitis (AD) is recognized as a multifactorial, heterogeneous disease characterized by different clinical phenotypes based on interactions of susceptibility genes, environmental factors, impaired skin barrier integrity, and immune dysregulation. Although barrier impairment and immune dysregulation play major roles in pathogenesis, their sequential order is unclear. The outside-in theory suggests that dysfunctional epidermal barrier incites the disease with secondary immunologic changes. Conversely, the inside-out hypothesis holds that immune dysregulation drives the disease and barrier changes are an epiphenomenon.[1] Recent genome-wide association studies identified loci correlated with autoimmune regulation, including genes associated with regulation of innate host defenses and T-cell function,[2] linking AD to other autoimmune or inflammatory diseases. Present treatments are limited and are not without adverse effects, creating a large unmet need for targeted approaches.[1]

This article highlights key advances in the understanding of AD pathophysiology, including immune dysregulation, skin barrier dysfunction, environmental, genetic, and microbiome effects, with implications for therapeutic interventions.

Disclosure Statement: The authors have nothing to disclose.
^a Department of Dermatology, Icahn School of Medicine at Mount Sinai, 1425 Madison Avenue, New York, NY 10029, USA; ^b Laboratory of Investigative Dermatology, The Rockefeller University, 1230 York Avenue, New York, NY 10065, USA; ^c SUNY Downstate College of Medicine, 450 Clarkson Avenue, Brooklyn, NY 11203, USA; ^d University of Maryland School of Medicine, 655 West Baltimore South, Baltimore, MD 21201, USA
¹ Present address: 169 Manhattan Avenue, #1D, New York, NY 10025.
² Present address: 777 South Eden Street, #1031, Baltimore, MD 21231.
* Corresponding author. Laboratory of Investigative Dermatology, The Rockefeller University, 1230 York Avenue, New York, NY 10065.
E-mail address: Tali.czarnowicki@mountsinai.org

Dermatol Clin 35 (2017) 317–326
http://dx.doi.org/10.1016/j.det.2017.02.006
0733-8635/17/© 2017 Elsevier Inc. All rights reserved.

IMMUNE DYSREGULATION

Dysregulation of both innate and adaptive immune systems are involved in AD. Although keratinocytes, antimicrobial peptides (AMPs), innate lymphoid cells group 2 (ILC-2), and toll-like receptors (TLRs) are major players of the innate arm, the discovery of T helper (Th) subsets Th17/Th22 has shed new light on the adaptive arm of AD pathogenesis, progressing from past models perceiving AD as a Th1/Th2 biphasic disease into the current concept of a multiple-cytokine axes disorder.

Although the pathogenetic role of autoimmunity in AD remains to be elucidated,[3] a recent meta-analysis reported autoimmune phenomenon in up to 91% of AD patients,[4] possibly a consequence of unrecognized self-epitopes.

Innate Immune System

Critical by virtue of their location, keratinocytes serve as sentinel cells with various downstream effects. AMPs, generated by keratinocytes, are divided into 2 classes: cathelicidin (LL-37) and human-β-defensins 2 and 3,[3] which play key roles in pathogen clearance and maintenance of tight junction integrity.[3] In AD skin, both subsets are reduced, contributing to increased infections.[5] AMPs induce several cytokines/chemokines, including interleukin (IL)-4, IL-13, IL-25, IL-33, and thymic stromal lymphopoietin (TSLP).[6] IL-25, IL-33, and TSLP affect dermal ILC-2 to produce IL-5 and IL-13.[6] ILC-2 increases and subsequent Th2 cytokine production, leads to Th2 axis augmentation in positive feedback loops.[7] Mutations in TLRs and nucleotide-binding oligomerization domain-like receptors (NLRs) also play roles in AD.[3] TLR2, which enhances tight junction integrity and defenses against Staphylococcus aureus and herpes simplex virus infections, shows decreased expression in AD.[8]

Adaptive Immune System

T helper-1

Expanded in chronic lesions,[9] Th1 has been shown in severe AD patients to have a skin selective or cutaneous lymphocyte antigen (CLA)-positive defect[10] which might potentially add to susceptibility for cutaneous infections. Ustekinumab, an IL-12/IL-23p40 antagonist, is currently being explored in clinical trials (Table 1). Mixed results have been documented, with some case reports showing clinical efficacy,[11] whereas others[12] demonstrated only limited benefit in clearing AD lesions. A recent phase II, double-blinded, placebo-controlled study[13] showed ustekinumab to modulate Th1, Th17,

Th22, and also Th2-related AD genes; however, there were no significant differences in clinical outcomes versus placebo. The interpretation of these results is limited due to the crossover study design, added to the effect of topical corticosteroids, which were allowed in all cohorts. A more recent study[14] of severe AD subjects found ustekinumab to reduce Eczema Area and Severity Index (EASI) by 50% at the end of treatment. In this study, ustekinumab also decreased epidermal hyperplasia or proliferation, dermal T-cell infiltrates, dendritic cells (DCs), and mast cells with quantitative polymerase chain reaction showing reduction in Th2/Th22 markers.[14] These conflicting results demand larger trials.

T helper-2

Increased Th2-related marker expression, including IL-5, IL-13, IL-10, IL-31, and chemokine (C-C motif) ligand (CCL)-5, CCL13, and CCL18, is prominent in acute lesions and augmented in chronic AD.[9] Th2 products downregulate AMP and epidermal differentiation complex (EDC) genes, thus suppressing major terminal differentiation proteins (filaggrin [FLG], loricrin [LOR], and involucrin [IVL]), whereas upregulating kallikreins (KLKs) are responsible for corneodesmosome degradation.[15] Th2 products permit antibody responses that include immunoglobulin (Ig)-E isotype-switching and mast cell or eosinophil differentiation,[9] though IgE itself is not a key mediator of AD pathogenesis.[16] IL-33/IL-31, involved in pruritus induction and in food allergies,[17] were found to be upregulated in AD lesional skin.[18] These new insights have led to active testing of immune axes-specific drugs. Dupilumab, an anti-IL-4Rα, has been shown to normalize Th2 inflammatory cytokines but also reverse barrier abnormalities, underlining the ongoing crosstalk between these 2 components (see Table 1).

T helper-9

Th9 cells are a relatively newly recognized skin-tropic T-cell subset[19] that are generated from naïve T cells (in the presence of transforming growth factor [TGF]-β and IL-4) or differentiated from Th2 cells.[20] Although Th9 cells are thought to be main producers of IL-9, which is elevated in AD skin lesions and sera of adults and children, the role of Th9/IL-9 in AD pathophysiology is obscure.[21–23] IL-9 functions to drive T-cell survival, proliferation, and secretion of inflammatory mediators, and seems to play a role in activation of ILCs, in which it enhances IL-5 and IL-13 production.[20] In keratinocytes, IL-9 induces VEGF,[24] which has been associated with epidermal changes seen in AD. Nonetheless, a genomic and molecular profiling of nonlesional, acute, and chronic AD

Table 1
Biologics in clinical trials for atopic dermatitis

Category or Targeted Axis	Target	Trade Name and ClinicalTrials.gov Identifier
Th1/Th17	Anti-IL-12/23 (anti-p40) mAb	Stelara (ustekinumab)/NCT01806662
	Anti-IL-17 mAb	Secukinumab/NCT02594098
Th2	Anti-IL-4Rα mAb	Dupilumab/NCT02260986
	Anti-IL-13 mAb	NCT02340234
		NCT02347176
	CRTH2 antagonist	NCT01785602
		NCT02002208
		NCT02590289
Th22	Anti-IL-22 mAb	ILV-094/NCT01941537
	TSLP antagonist	Tezepelumab/NCT02525094
PDE4 inhibitors		Otezla (Apremilast)/NCT02087943
		NCT01856764
		NCT01461941
		NCT02094235
		NCT02068352
		NCT01993420
		NCT01037881
		Crisaborole/NCT02118792
		NCT02118766
Antipruritic	Anti-IL-31 mAb	NCT01986933
		NCT01614756
	Antitropomyosin receptor kinase A	NCT01808157
	Antineurokinin	NCT02004041
		NCT01033097
	Prostaglandin D2 receptor agonist	NCT00914186
	Anti-TRPV1 channel	NCT02583022
	Kappa-opioid receptor agonist	NCT02475447
		NCT02576093

Abbreviations: CRTH2, chemokine receptor homologous molecule expressed on Th2 lymphocytes; mAb, monoclonal antibodies; PDE4, phophodiesterase 4; TRPV1, transient receptor potential cation channel subfamily V member 1; TSLP, thymic stromal lymphopoietin.

lesions[9] showed no significant difference in IL-9 levels between these tissues, though acute and chronic lesions had similar increases in IL-9 levels compared with nonlesional skin. Other studies show IL-9 levels in skin and in serum to correlate with Scoring Atopic Dermatitis (SCORAD), serum IgE, and CCL17 levels.[24] However, the relevance of Th9/IL-9 in AD pathogenesis remains incompletely understood and is only beginning elucidation.

T helper-22
Th22 and associated markers are upregulated in acute AD with intensification in chronic lesions.[9] IL-22 was reported to correlate with disease severity,[6] induce epidermal hyperplasia, inhibit terminal differentiation, and regulate skin barrier function.[25] Drugs targeting the Th22 axis are actively undergoing phase II trials (see **Table 1**).

T helper-17
The Th17 immune axis is generally attenuated in AD,[9] though some studies report it being increased.[26] Although the role of Th17 T cells in AD remains controversial, it is thought that the robust Th2 cytokine signal seen in AD inhibits the Th17 axis.[27] IL-17 has been shown to infiltrate AD lesions, modify epithelial cells and keratinocytes to produce inflammatory cytokines,[28] and downregulate filaggrin and other epidermal barrier gene expressions.[29] Anti-IL17 phase II trials are ongoing (see **Table 1**).

Dendritic Cells
CD11+ myeloid DCs (mDCs), are found in chronic lesions.[15] Other DC subtypes include plasmacytoid DCs, increased in chronic AD, and blood DC antigen positive and CD123+ DCs, which secrete interferon (IFN)-α and mediate lesion formation.[15]

Inflammatory dendritic epidermal DCs (IDECs), a type of mDC, are important contributors to T-cell activation.[30] Dermal DCs (dDCs), which express the same markers as IDECs, are localized to the dermis and have important immunostimulatory effects in acute AD.[30] dDCs express high levels of TSLP, which induces a Th1/Th17 response and Th2 polarization through various chemoattractants (CCL17, CCL 22, CCL24) in an OX40-dependent mechanism.[15]

Regulatory T cells

Reports[31] show increased regulatory T cell (Treg) counts in AD lesions, and serum Treg levels to positively correlate with disease severity. However, the exact role of Tregs in AD remains to be clarified.[15]

Finally, increased activity of phosphodiesterase (PDE) activity was implicated in AD, reducing Th1 and enhancing Th2 signals. Inhibition of PDE4, located in keratinocytes and a wide variety of immune cells, increases levels of cAMP, leading to inhibition of proinflammatory cytokines.[32] PDE4 inhibition by apremilast and crisaborole, have shown to be efficacious (see **Table 1**).[6]

Certain patient groups show distinct immune responses, supporting the complex molecular and cellular phenotype characterizing AD. Asian AD is Th17 polarized,[33] whereas intrinsic AD has more robust immune activation and a significantly increased Th17 signal.[34] Pediatric AD is characterized by a multi-axes activation in skin lesions[35] but only Th2/Th1 imbalance in blood.[35] These findings implicate tailored strategies that target distinct phenotypes.

SKIN BARRIER

The epidermal barrier prevents allergen penetration, maintains skin hydration, and displays antimicrobial activity, while having an ongoing interaction with the adaptive immune system.[1] The barrier is composed of a complex matrix of structural proteins and lipids held together by desmosomes and tight junctions.[36] Deficiency of these components, lack of keratinocyte differentiation, and immune dysregulation are the basis for barrier dysfunction in AD.[37]

Filaggrin

The skin barrier is composed of a cornified envelope (CE), essential for barrier function. The CE is composed of terminally differentiated keratinocytes, structural proteins (LOR, IVL, and FLG), and lipids.[1] FLG is a structural protein important for cornification, skin hydration, and AMP function.[37] FLG mutations are strongly associated with AD but are found only in 15% to 50% of patients.[38] Additionally, approximately 40% of FLG mutations carriers never develop AD.[38] FLG deficiency is associated with early onset, severe AD, greater allergen sensitization, and increased susceptibility to infections.[39] FLG degradation products are components of the natural moisturizing factor (NMF), vital for skin hydration.[40] Lower levels of NMF and greater transepidermal water loss (TEWL) have been observed in AD patients with FLG mutations.[40]

LIPIDS

Lesional and nonlesional AD skin is characterized by reduced ceramide composition, as well as reduced ceramide to cholesterol ratios,[41] alterations which lead to increased TEWL. Cole and colleagues[42] performed a meta-analysis to define the AD transcriptome showing abnormalities in lipid metabolism genes despite normal FLG genes. Additionally, Th2 activation correlated with downregulation of key epidermal lipids.[43] Ceramide-dominant moisturizers have shown to restore integrity of the skin barrier.[44] A recent evidence-based review evaluating the efficacy of topical or oral oils concluded that topical sunflower seed or coconut oil may be potential therapies for AD[45]; however, larger, well-designed studies are needed.

Tight Junctions

Tight junctions, transmembrane proteins regulating the permeability of the epidermis, are decreased in AD.[46] Claudins are tight junction proteins found on keratinocytes that further strengthen the epidermal barrier. Claudin1 gene expression is downregulated in AD, and shown to negatively correlate with Th2 cytokines, serum IgE, and serum eosinophils.[46] Yuki and colleagues[47] reported that impaired tight junctions affect lipids and FLG processing by disturbing skin pH. TLR2 activation, reduced in AD, has been shown to increase expression of tight junction proteins and enhance barrier function.[8]

Skin pH

An acidic skin pH (4–6) is necessary to maintain the integrity of the stratum corneum, lipid metabolism, epidermal differentiation, and antimicrobial functions.[48] The baseline skin pH in AD is high.[49] FLG deficiency may contribute to this increased pH due to decreased acidic FLG breakdown products.[37] Increased pH enhances serine protease activity in the stratum corneum. Jang and colleagues[50] evaluated the role of pH in AD

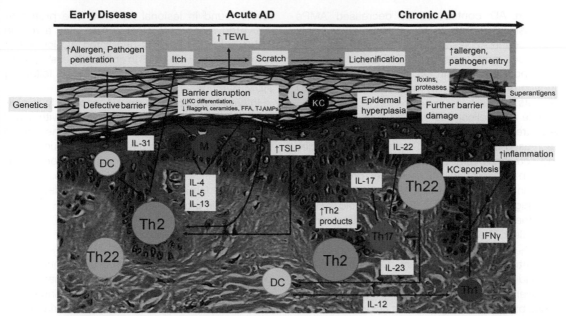

Fig. 1. Defective skin barrier allows for allergen or pathogen penetration, activating DCs to induce Th2 proliferation. Th2 cells produce cytokines that disrupt expression of structural proteins and impair lipid production, resulting in further barrier disruption and reduced skin hydration in acute lesions. Mast cells (M) and eosinophils (E) activated by Th2 cytokines release factors contributing to pruritus and inflammation. IL-31, a Th2 cytokine, contributes to pruritus, which perpetuates barrier disruption. Activated keratinocytes (KCs) induce TSLP expression, amplifying Th2 responses. In chronic disease, intensified Th22 responses contribute to epidermal hyperplasia and continued barrier dysfunction. Activation of interferon (IFN)-γ producing Th1 cells results in increased inflammation, KC apoptosis, and barrier damage. In chronic AD, weakened barrier permits ongoing allergen or pathogen penetration and continued damage to the skin directly, as well as indirectly through immune activation. AMPs, antimicrobial peptides; FFA, free fatty acids; LC, Langerhans cells; TJ, tight junctions.

pathogenesis and found that in mice, skin alkalinization-induced KLK5 led to skin barrier dysfunction, pruritus, and dermatitis. The increased activity of serine proteases leads to over-degradation of structural proteins and lipids, and decreased barrier integrity.[51] Acidic pH inhibits the growth of pathogens such as S aureus, and decreases the expression of staphylococcal surface-binding proteins.[37] Thus, alkaline pH in AD promotes bacterial growth, contributing to an altered skin microbial profile.

Skin barrier plays a major role in AD pathogenesis, making it an attractive prophylactic and therapeutic target. Early use of emollients can prevent AD in 50% of high-risk infants,[52] highlighting the critical role barrier integrity plays in AD initiation.

The interplay between barrier integrity and immune dysregulation is complex (**Fig. 1**). For example, Th2 and Th22 downregulate EDC gene expression, suppress terminal differentiation, inhibit desmoglein 3 expression and ceramide synthesis, modulate FLG expression, and induce epidermal hyperplasia.[53] Additionally, correction of the barrier ameliorates inflammation, reinforcing this concept.[53]

SKIN MICROBIOME

Commensal S epidermidis plays a protective role by producing AMPs and proteases, preventing the growth of pathogenic species, and limiting S aureus biofilm formation.[5] AD skin exhibits a decrease in overall microbial diversity.[54] Loss of microbial diversity leading to S aureus dominance occurs shortly before AD flares.[55] S aureus plays a critical role in AD. Nakatsuji and colleagues[56] demonstrated that S aureus penetration across the epidermis directly correlated with increased IL-4, IL-13, IL-22, and TSLP, and decreased expression of AMPs.[56] S aureus superantigens have been shown to increase Th2 inflammation.[56] Th2 cytokines enhance the susceptibility of keratinocytes to S aureus alpha toxin toxicity.[57]

S aureus colonization is detectable in greater than 90% of AD skin compared with approximately 10% of controls.[58] The complex interaction between an impaired skin barrier, immune dysregulation, FLG mutations, and an altered skin microbiome contributes to increased infection susceptibility in AD. IL-17 is a known inducer of AMPs in keratinocytes.[59] Relatively reduced

IL-17 in AD contributes to decreased AMPs expression.[60] TSLP, a Th2-related marker highly expressed in AD lesions, may also promote AMP decreases and subsequent increased infection predisposition. Vitamin D3, which enhances production of AMPs in skin, may be beneficial in AD patients.[61]

Seite and colleagues[62] found successful emollient treatment in AD to be associated with decreased abundance of Staphylococcal species and increased overall bacterial diversity. The administration of lactobacillus and other probiotics to pregnant women decreased the risk of developing AD in high-risk infants by half at 2 years old.[63] However, the effectiveness of probiotics as treatment is still unclear. The use of antimicrobial treatment in AD patients without clinical evidence of superinfection is controversial.[64] A recent Cochrane review concluded no clinical benefit of antimicrobial therapy over topical anti-inflammatory agents and antiseptic baths in treating S aureus colonization.[64]

ENVIRONMENTAL FACTORS

More than 85% of AD patients are IgE sensitized to house dust mite (HDM).[3] Added to the seasonal variation characterizing AD, environmental agents are thought to play a role in disease pathogenesis.[3] Although the exact role of airborne allergens in AD remains controversial, a recent double-blinded, placebo-controlled trial demonstrated grass-allergen-sensitized adults with AD exposed to grass pollen to have worsening of their cutaneous symptoms, with elevated serum IL-4 and CCL17/22 levels, indicating a Th2 response.[65] In children, food allergens may play a role in AD flares.[3] Allergen patterns shift with aging, including inhalant allergens in adulthood. More than 85% of sensitized adults have specific IgEs to HDM, though most do not have clinical allergy.[3]

Even in patients without elevated IgE or clinical allergy, HDM can be problematic because it is known to trigger AD-like lesions through nonallergic mechanisms. Treatment of a human keratinocyte line with HDM extract for 48 and 72 hours showed HDM to increase keratinocyte proliferation.[66] In this same study, HDM increased expression of IL-22Rα and CCL17/thymus and activation-regulated chemokine (TARC) in the keratinocyte line, as well as increasing IL-22 production from T cells.[66] Other studies[67,68] have shown the major allergen of HDM, the cysteine protease Der p1, to directly induce TSLP expression in vitro in human bronchial epithelial cells. In vivo studies[69] in nonlesional skin of AD subjects show epicutaneous application of HDM to induce TSLP and CCL17/TARC expression, comparable to

levels found in lesional AD skin. The protease-activated receptor-2 (PAR-2) may play a role in TSLP induction in HDM-generated AD lesions (it is known to induce TSLP in epithelial cells[68]); however, PAR-2 expression did not change following HDM patch testing in this study.[69]

Influences of climate on AD, especially in children, show lower disease prevalence with lower precipitation, less indoor heating, higher mean temperatures, and higher relative humidity.[70] Other established environmental factors influencing AD include use of alkaline soaps, western diet, small family size, high education level, and residence in urban settings.[71]

GENETICS

Genome-wide association and single-nucleotide polymorphism studies have identified many gene susceptibility loci in AD patients.[2] An increased risk of AD has been associated with variations in genes involved in skin barrier function, keratinocyte differentiation, innate and adaptive immune responses, and cytokines and chemokines.[2] FLG mutations (mostly loss-of-function) are most consistently associated with AD.[72] FLG gene copy number variation influences the risk of developing AD in a dose-dependent manner.[72] Other genes involved in skin barrier function include those encoding structural and tight junction proteins.[46] Recently, a polymorphism of Tmem79/matt gene, which encodes for lamellar granular proteins required for lipid processing, proteases, and AMPs, has been found to be associated with AD in humans.[73]

Polymorphisms and mutations in genes encoding serine proteases and serine protease inhibitors have also been associated with AD.[74] The serine protease inhibitor Kazal-type 5 (SPINK5) gene encodes lymphoepithelial Kazal-type–related inhibitor (LEKTI), which is expressed in the epithelium and regulates proteolysis of keratinocyte differentiation and maintenance of the normal skin barrier.[75] Although SPINK5 mutations are known to be associated with Netherton syndrome, recent studies have linked them with AD.[76] Mutations in AMPs and in pattern-recognition receptors (PRR) such as TLRs and NLRs, have been associated with AD and the increased susceptibility to infections.[75] Mutations and polymorphisms of various cytokine/chemokine genes have found to increase disease risk in certain populations.[75]

ITCH-SCRATCH CYCLE

Pruritus is a primary feature of AD. The itch-scratch cycle promotes further inflammation through release of mediators (TSLP, IL-13, and IL-31) that stimulate nerve fibers and upregulate cellular pruritogens.[71] Although the exact mechanisms of pruritus are elusive, processes at epidermal and neuronal levels are involved, including increased epidermal proteases, increased PAR-2 responsiveness, and release of skin-damaging neuromediators.[77] Communication between keratinocytes and immune cells is important in itch regulation because these cells generate mediators that contribute to sprouting of nerve fibers and stimulate sensory nerve endings.[71] Recently, human sensory neurons have shown to express IL-31R and signal in response to IL-31, a process that is transient receptor channel potential cation channel ankyrin subtype 1 (TRPA1)-dependent in model systems.[78] TRPA1 is known to be an important intermediary for histamine-independent, bradykinin-mediated itch.[78]

Breaking the itch-scratch cycle is crucial to prevent AD progression. IL-31, TSLP, and CRTH2 (chemokine receptor homologous molecule expressed on Th2 lymphocytes) antagonists, as well as other agents, are currently being evaluated as anti-itch treatment (see **Table 1**).[6]

SUMMARY

AD is a complex, multifactorial disease. Immune dysregulation, barrier impairment, microbial shifts, environmental factors, and genetic propensity all orchestrate the disease phenotype. This is a very exciting era in AD research because accumulating mechanistic studies are now enabling identification of novel key mediators and mechanisms that drive and perpetuate AD. With the current limited armamentarium of topical and systemic therapies that harbor toxic effects, the need for novel targeted treatments is at its greatest. As key advances in the understanding of AD continue to be made, efficacious, safe, and targeted treatments, along with preventive measures, may provide promising outcomes to affected individuals.

REFERENCES

1. Leung DY. Clinical implications of new mechanistic insights into atopic dermatitis. Curr Opin Pediatr 2016;28:456–62.
2. Paternoster L, Standl M, Waage J, et al. Multi-ethnic genome-wide association study of 21,000 cases and 95,000 controls identifies new risk loci for atopic dermatitis. Nat Genet 2015;47:1449.
3. D'Auria E, Banderali G, Barberi S, et al. Atopic dermatitis: recent insight on pathogenesis and novel therapeutic target. Asian Pac J Allergy Immunol 2016;34:98–108.
4. Tang TS, Bieber T, Williams HC. Does "autoreactivity" play a role in atopic dermatitis? J Allergy Clin Immunol 2012;129:1209–15.e2.
5. Williams MR, Gallo RL. The role of the skin microbiome in atopic dermatitis. Curr Allergy Asthma Rep 2015;15:65.
6. Wang D, Beck LA. Immunologic targets in atopic dermatitis and emerging therapies: an update. Am J Clin Dermatol 2016;17(5):425–43.
7. Mjosberg J, Eidsmo L. Update on innate lymphoid cells in atopic and nonatopic inflammation in the airways and skin. Clin Exp Allergy 2014;44:1033–43.
8. Kuo IH, Carpenter-Mendini A, Yoshida T, et al. Activation of epidermal toll-like receptor 2 enhances tight junction function: implications for atopic dermatitis and skin barrier repair. J Invest Dermatol 2013;133:988–98.
9. Gittler JK, Shemer A, Suarez-Farinas M, et al. Progressive activation of T(H)2/T(H)22 cytokines and selective epidermal proteins characterizes acute and chronic atopic dermatitis. J Allergy Clin Immunol 2012;130:1344–54.
10. Czarnowicki T, Gonzalez J, Shemer A, et al. Severe atopic dermatitis is characterized by selective expansion of circulating TH2/TC2 and TH22/TC22, but not TH17/TC17, cells within the skin-homing T-cell population. J Allergy Clin Immunol 2015;136:104–15.e7.
11. Shroff A, Guttman-Yassky E. Successful use of ustekinumab therapy in refractory severe atopic dermatitis. JAAD Case Rep 2015;1:25–6.
12. Samorano LP, Hanifin JM, Simpson EL, et al. Inadequate response to ustekinumab in atopic dermatitis - a report of two patients. J Eur Acad Dermatol Venereol 2016;30:522–3.
13. Khattri S, Brunner PM, Garcet S, et al. Efficacy and safety of ustekinumab treatment in adults with moderate-to-severe atopic dermatitis. Exp Dermatol 2016;26(1):28–35.
14. Weiss D, Schaschinger M, Ristl R, et al. Ustekinumab treatment in severe atopic dermatitis: downregulation of T-helper 2/22 expression. J Am Acad Dermatol 2016;76(1):91–7.e3.
15. Guttman-Yassky E, Nograles KE, Krueger JG. Contrasting pathogenesis of atopic dermatitis and psoriasis–part II: immune cell subsets and therapeutic concepts. J Allergy Clin Immunol 2011;127:1420–32.
16. Guttman-Yassky E, Nograles KE, Krueger JG. Contrasting pathogenesis of atopic dermatitis and psoriasis–part I: clinical and pathologic concepts. J Allergy Clin Immunol 2011;127:1110–8.
17. Saluja R, Khan M, Church MK, et al. The role of IL-33 and mast cells in allergy and inflammation. Clin Transl Allergy 2015;5:33.
18. Balato A, Lembo S, Mattii M, et al. IL-33 is secreted by psoriatic keratinocytes and induces

pro-inflammatory cytokines via keratinocyte and mast cell activation. Exp Dermatol 2012;21:892–4.

19. Wang AX, Xu Landen N. New insights into T cells and their signature cytokines in atopic dermatitis. IUBMB Life 2015;67:601–10.

20. Clark RA, Schlapbach C. TH9 cells in skin disorders. Semin Immunopathol 2016;39(1):47–54.

21. Berker M, Frank LJ, Gessner AL, et al. Allergies - A T cells perspective in the era beyond the TH1/TH2 paradigm. Clin Immunol 2016;174:73–83.

22. Esaki H, Brunner PM, Renert-Yuval Y, et al. Early-onset pediatric atopic dermatitis is TH2 but also TH17 polarized in skin. J Allergy Clin Immunol 2016;138(6):1639–51.

23. Ciprandi G, De Amici M, Giunta V, et al. Serum interleukin-9 levels are associated with clinical severity in children with atopic dermatitis. Pediatr Dermatol 2013;30:222–5.

24. Ma L, Xue HB, Guan XH, et al. Possible pathogenic role of T helper type 9 cells and interleukin (IL)-9 in atopic dermatitis. Clin Exp Immunol 2014;175: 25–31.

25. Nograles KE, Zaba LC, Guttman-Yassky E, et al. Th17 cytokines interleukin (IL)-17 and IL-22 modulate distinct inflammatory and keratinocyte-response pathways. Br J Dermatol 2008;159:1092–102.

26. Clausen ML, Jungersted JM, Andersen PS, et al. Human beta-defensin-2 as a marker for disease severity and skin barrier properties in atopic dermatitis. Br J Dermatol 2013;169:587–93.

27. Howell MD, Fairchild HR, Kim BE, et al. Th2 cytokines act on S100/A11 to downregulate keratinocyte differentiation. J Invest Dermatol 2008;128:2248–58.

28. Kabashima-Kubo R, Nakamura M, Sakabe J, et al. A group of atopic dermatitis without IgE elevation or barrier impairment shows a high Th1 frequency: possible immunological state of the intrinsic type. J Dermatol Sci 2012;67:37–43.

29. Gutowska-Owsiak D, Schaupp AL, Salimi M, et al. IL-17 downregulates filaggrin and affects keratinocyte expression of genes associated with cellular adhesion. Exp Dermatol 2012;21:104–10.

30. Novak N, Koch S, Allam JP, et al. Dendritic cells: bridging innate and adaptive immunity in atopic dermatitis. J Allergy Clin Immunol 2010;125:50–9.

31. Moosbrugger-Martinz V, Tripp CH, Clausen BE, et al. Atopic dermatitis induces the expansion of thymus-derived regulatory T cells exhibiting a Th2-like phenotype in mice. J Cell Mol Med 2016;20:930–8.

32. Saporito RC, Cohen DJ. Apremilast use for moderate-to-severe atopic dermatitis in pediatric patients. Case Rep Dermatol 2016;8:179–84.

33. Noda S, Suarez-Farinas M, Ungar B, et al. The Asian atopic dermatitis phenotype combines features of atopic dermatitis and psoriasis with increased TH17 polarization. J Allergy Clin Immunol 2015; 136:1254–64.

34. Suarez-Farinas M, Dhingra N, Gittler J, et al. Intrinsic atopic dermatitis shows similar TH2 and higher TH17 immune activation compared with extrinsic atopic dermatitis. J Allergy Clin Immunol 2013;132: 361–70.

35. Czarnowicki T, Esaki H, Gonzalez J, et al. Early pediatric atopic dermatitis shows only a cutaneous lymphocyte antigen (CLA)(+) TH2/TH1 cell imbalance, whereas adults acquire CLA(+) TH22/TC22 cell subsets. J Allergy Clin Immunol 2015;136:941–51.e3.

36. Yu HS, Kang MJ, Kwon JW, et al. Claudin-1 polymorphism modifies the effect of mold exposure on the development of atopic dermatitis and production of IgE. J Allergy Clin Immunol 2015;135:827–30.e5.

37. Lee HJ, Lee SH. Epidermal permeability barrier defects and barrier repair therapy in atopic dermatitis. Allergy Asthma Immunol Res 2014;6:276–87.

38. Palmer CN, Irvine AD, Terron-Kwiatkowski A, et al. Common loss-of-function variants of the epidermal barrier protein filaggrin are a major predisposing factor for atopic dermatitis. Nat Genet 2006;38: 441–6.

39. Szegedi A. Filaggrin mutations in early- and late-onset atopic dermatitis. Br J Dermatol 2015;172: 320–1.

40. Riethmuller C, McAleer MA, Koppes SA, et al. Filaggrin breakdown products determine corneocyte conformation in patients with atopic dermatitis. J Allergy Clin Immunol 2015;136:1573–80.e1-2.

41. Jungersted JM, Scheer H, Mempel M, et al. Stratum corneum lipids, skin barrier function and filaggrin mutations in patients with atopic eczema. Allergy 2010;65:911–8.

42. Cole C, Kroboth K, Schurch NJ, et al. Filaggrin-stratified transcriptomic analysis of pediatric skin identifies mechanistic pathways in patients with atopic dermatitis. J Allergy Clin Immunol 2014; 134:82–91.

43. Ewald DA, Malajian D, Krueger JG, et al. Meta-analysis derived atopic dermatitis (MADAD) transcriptome defines a robust AD signature highlighting the involvement of atherosclerosis and lipid metabolism pathways. BMC Med Genomics 2015;8:60.

44. Sajic D, Asiniwasis R, Skotnicki-Grant S. A look at epidermal barrier function in atopic dermatitis: physiologic lipid replacement and the role of ceramides. Skin Therapy Lett 2012;17:6–9.

45. Vieira BL, Lim NR, Lohman ME, et al. Complementary and alternative medicine for atopic dermatitis: an evidence-based review. Am J Clin Dermatol 2016;17(6):557–81.

46. De Benedetto A, Rafaels NM, McGirt LY, et al. Tight junction defects in patients with atopic dermatitis. J Allergy Clin Immunol 2011;127:773–86.e1-7.

47. Yuki T, Komiya A, Kusaka A, et al. Impaired tight junctions obstruct stratum corneum formation by

altering polar lipid and profilaggrin processing. J Dermatol Sci 2013;69:148–58.

48. Ali SM, Yosipovitch G. Skin pH: from basic science to basic skin care. Acta Derm Venereol 2013;93: 261–7.

49. Eberlein-Konig B, Schafer T, Huss-Marp J, et al. Skin surface pH, stratum corneum hydration, transepidermal water loss and skin roughness related to atopic eczema and skin dryness in a population of primary school children. Acta Derm Venereol 2000; 80:188–91.

50. Jang H, Matsuda A, Jung K, et al. Skin pH is the master switch of kallikrein 5-mediated skin barrier destruction in a murine atopic dermatitis model. J Invest Dermatol 2016;136:127–35.

51. Lee SE, Jeong SK, Lee SH. Protease and protease-activated receptor-2 signaling in the pathogenesis of atopic dermatitis. Yonsei Med J 2010;51:808–22.

52. Horimukai K, Morita K, Narita M, et al. Application of moisturizer to neonates prevents development of atopic dermatitis. J Allergy Clin Immunol 2014;134: 824–30.e6.

53. Czarnowicki T, Krueger JG, Guttman-Yassky E. Skin barrier and immune dysregulation in atopic dermatitis: an evolving story with important clinical implications. J Allergy Clin Immunol Pract 2014;2:371–9 [quiz: 380–1].

54. Tauber M, Balica S, Hsu CY, et al. Staphylococcus aureus density on lesional and nonlesional skin is strongly associated with disease severity in atopic dermatitis. J Allergy Clin Immunol 2016;137:1272–4. e1-3.

55. Kong HH, Oh J, Deming C, et al. Temporal shifts in the skin microbiome associated with disease flares and treatment in children with atopic dermatitis. Genome Res 2012;22:850–9.

56. Nakatsuji T, Chen TH, Two AM, et al. Staphylococcus aureus exploits epidermal barrier defects in atopic dermatitis to trigger cytokine expression. J Invest Dermatol 2016;136(11):2192–200.

57. Brauweiler AM, Goleva E, Leung DY. Th2 cytokines increase Staphylococcus aureus alpha toxin-induced keratinocyte death through the signal transducer and activator of transcription 6 (STAT6). J Invest Dermatol 2014;134:2114–21.

58. Ong PY. Recurrent MRSA skin infections in atopic dermatitis. J Allergy Clin Immunol Pract 2014;2: 396–9.

59. Nograles KE, Zaba LC, Shemer A, et al. IL-22-producing "T22" T cells account for upregulated IL-22 in atopic dermatitis despite reduced IL-17-producing TH17 T cells. J Allergy Clin Immunol 2009;123:1244–52.e2.

60. Wolk K, Mitsui H, Witte K, et al. Deficient cutaneous antibacterial competence in cutaneous T-cell lymphomas: role of Th2-mediated biased Th17 function. Clin Cancer Res 2014;20:5507–16.

61. van der Does AM, Kenne E, Koppelaar E, et al. Vitamin D(3) and phenylbutyrate promote development of a human dendritic cell subset displaying enhanced antimicrobial properties. J Leukoc Biol 2014;95:883–91.

62. Seite S, Flores GE, Henley JB, et al. Microbiome of affected and unaffected skin of patients with atopic dermatitis before and after emollient treatment. J Drugs Dermatol 2014;13:1365–72.

63. Panduru M, Panduru NM, Salavastru CM, et al. Probiotics and primary prevention of atopic dermatitis: a meta-analysis of randomized controlled studies. J Eur Acad Dermatol Venereol 2015;29:232–42.

64. Bath-Hextall FJ, Birnie AJ, Ravenscroft JC, et al. Interventions to reduce Staphylococcus aureus in the management of atopic eczema: an updated Cochrane review. Br J Dermatol 2010;163:12–26.

65. Werfel T, Heratizadeh A, Niebuhr M, et al. Exacerbation of atopic dermatitis on grass pollen exposure in an environmental challenge chamber. J Allergy Clin Immunol 2015;136:96–103.e9.

66. Jang M, Kim H, Kim Y, et al. The crucial role of IL-22 and its receptor in thymus and activation regulated chemokine production and T-cell migration by house dust mite extract. Exp Dermatol 2016;25: 598–603.

67. Al-Ghouleh A, Johal R, Sharquie IK, et al. The glycosylation pattern of common allergens: the recognition and uptake of Der p 1 by epithelial and dendritic cells is carbohydrate dependent. PLoS One 2012;7:e33929.

68. Kouzaki H, O'Grady SM, Lawrence CB, et al. Proteases induce production of thymic stromal lymphopoietin by airway epithelial cells through protease-activated receptor-2. J Immunol 2009; 183:1427–34.

69. Landheer J, Giovannone B, Mattson JD, et al. Epicutaneous application of house dust mite induces thymic stromal lymphopoietin in nonlesional skin of patients with atopic dermatitis. J Allergy Clin Immunol 2013;132:1252–4.

70. Totri CR, Diaz L, Eichenfield LF. 2014 update on atopic dermatitis in children. Curr Opin Pediatr 2014;26:466–71.

71. Weidinger S, Novak N. Atopic dermatitis. Lancet 2016;387:1109–22.

72. Brown SJ, Kroboth K, Sandilands A, et al. Intragenic copy number variation within filaggrin contributes to the risk of atopic dermatitis with a dose-dependent effect. J Invest Dermatol 2012;132:98–104.

73. Saunders SP, Goh CS, Brown SJ, et al. Tmem79/Matt is the matted mouse gene and is a predisposing gene for atopic dermatitis in human subjects. J Allergy Clin Immunol 2013;132:1121–9.

74. Oyoshi MK, He R, Kumar L, et al. Cellular and molecular mechanisms in atopic dermatitis. Adv Immunol 2009;102:135–226.

75. Mu Z, Zhao Y, Liu X, et al. Molecular biology of atopic dermatitis. Clin Rev Allergy Immunol 2014; 47:193–218.

76. Kato A, Fukai K, Oiso N, et al. Association of SPINK5 gene polymorphisms with atopic dermatitis in the Japanese population. Br J Dermatol 2003;148: 665–9.

77. Silverberg NB. A practical overview of pediatric atopic dermatitis, part 1: epidemiology and pathogenesis. Cutis 2016;97:267–71.

78. Lyons JJ, Milner JD, Stone KD. Atopic dermatitis in children: clinical features, pathophysiology, and treatment. Immunol Allergy Clin North Am 2015;35: 161–83.

The Role of Interleukins 4 and/or 13 in the Pathophysiology and Treatment of Atopic Dermatitis

CrossMark

Jonathan I. Silverberg, MD, PhD, MPH[a,b,c,*], Robert Kantor, MD[d]

KEYWORDS

- Atopic dermatitis • Eczema • Inflammation • T helper 2 • Interleukin 4 • Interleukin 13 • Biologic

KEY POINTS

- Atopic dermatitis is an inflammatory skin disease mediated by increased T helper 2 inflammation in the skin and blood.
- Novel biologics targeting the T helper 2 cytokines, interleukins 4 and 13, show promise for the treatment of moderate to severe atopic dermatitis.

INTRODUCTION

Atopic dermatitis (AD) is a chronic, pruritic, inflammatory skin and potentially multisystem disorder that is associated with considerable morbidity. The most common morbidity, severe itch, in AD may result in difficulty falling asleep, staying asleep, more frequent nighttime awakenings, nocturnal scratching, and poor sleep efficiency, ultimately leading to daytime fatigue and impairment of instrumental activities of daily living.[1–3] AD is also associated with increased symptoms of anxiety and depression and higher rates of diagnosed depression, anxiety, attention-deficit (hyperactivity) disorder, and other mental health disorders in both children and adults.[4–6] Moreover, chronic itch and AD are associated with impaired productivity at school and work, social and relationship problems, and poor health-related quality of life.[3,7,8]

AD is commonly associated with several atopic disorders in children and adults, including asthma, hay fever, and food allergy.[1,9] The overlap of these disorders suggests potentially overlapping disease mechanisms and/or triggers that extend beyond the skin. Recent studies have identified several previously unrecognized comorbidities of AD, including cardiovascular disease, myocardial infarction, stroke, obesity, osteoporosis, injury and fracture, alopecia areata, and vitiligo.[5,10–15] Taken together, the comorbid health conditions occurring in patients with AD suggest that AD is a systemic disease, with widespread harmful effects.

Dr J.I. Silverberg is a consultant for Abbvie, Anacor, GlaxoSmithKline, Lilly, Pfizer, Proctor & Gamble, MedImmune, and Regeneron-Sanofi.

[a] Department of Dermatology, Northwestern University Feinberg School of Medicine, 676 North St. Clair Street, Suite 1600, Chicago, IL 60611, USA; [b] Department of Preventive Medicine, Northwestern University Feinberg School of Medicine, 676 North St. Clair Street, Suite 1600, Chicago, IL 60611, USA; [c] Department of Medical Social Sciences, Northwestern University Feinberg School of Medicine, 676 North St. Clair Street, Suite 1600, Chicago, IL 60611, USA; [d] Department of Dermatology, Northwestern University Feinberg School of Medicine, 676 North St. Clair Street, Suite 1600, Chicago, IL 60611, USA
* Corresponding author. Department of Dermatology, Northwestern University Feinberg School of Medicine, 676 North St. Clair Street, Suite 1600, Chicago, IL 60611.
E-mail address: JonathanISilverberg@Gmail.com

Dermatol Clin 35 (2017) 327–334
http://dx.doi.org/10.1016/j.det.2017.02.005
0733-8635/17/© 2017 Elsevier Inc. All rights reserved.

There are currently several unmet needs in the management of AD, particularly pruritus.[16,17] First, AD is typically managed by treating flares after activity has become full blown. Although this approach is reasonable in patients with only occasional flares, it is inadequate in patients with frequent flares or persistent disease with daily symptoms. In fact, moderate AD may be associated with symptoms 1 out of every 3 days in perpetuity.[18] Second, AD is typically managed using topical therapies, including emollients, corticosteroids (TCS), and calcineurin inhibitors. Topical therapies are typically effective for treating mild disease, but may not be effective in more severe disease and do not address underlying systemic inflammation.[19] Moreover, they are impractical and difficult to apply for patients with extensive disease. Several systemic immunosuppressants have been shown to be effective for treating AD, including intramuscular or oral corticosteroids, cyclosporine, methotrexate, azathioprine, and to a lesser extent, mycophenolate mofetil.[20] Each of these agents has a poor adverse-effect and/or tolerability profile, which limits their use in the clinical dermatology setting and requires laboratory monitoring for adverse effects. For example, systemic corticosteroids can cause glucose intolerance, weight gain, insomnia, depression, psychosis, and adrenal and immune suppression. Cyclosporine can cause, among other side effects, headaches, anemia, nephrotoxicity, hypertension, hirsutism, and electrolyte abnormalities. Methotrexate can cause anemia, leukopenia, gastrointestinal discomfort, weakness, and hepatotoxicity. Even when these agents are successfully used for treating AD, their potential toxicity precludes them from being used long term. The US Food and Drug Administration (FDA) has recommended that cyclosporine not be used in other disorders more than 1 year. Moreover, none of these agents are approved by the FDA for the treatment of AD. Only cyclosporine is approved for the treatment of AD in Europe.

Improved understanding of the immune basis of disease has allowed for the development of multiple novel targeted therapies in the AD pipeline. The principal benefit of more targeted therapy is the combination of improved efficacy and safety. The treatment of moderate to severe psoriasis has been revolutionized by the advent of multiple biologic therapies.[21] This review focuses on the roles of interleukin 4 (IL-4) and/or -13 in the pathophysiology of and development of targeted biologics for AD.

PATHOGENESIS

AD pathophysiology involves the interaction of epidermal barrier dysfunction with systemic inflammation and immune dysregulation. However, a fundamental debate exists as to whether AD is driven primarily by barrier dysfunction (outside-inside hypothesis) or primarily by an inflammatory response to irritants and environmental allergens (inside-outside hypothesis).[22]

Outside-In Hypothesis

The "outside-in" hypothesis posits that epidermal barrier dysfunction precedes AD and is required for the disease to manifest.[23] The outside-in hypothesis is supported by previous studies demonstrating loss-of-function mutations in the filaggrin gene (FLG).[24] Suboptimal filaggrin proteins may alter epidermal corneocyte shape and change the organization of lamellar bodies, resulting in impaired barrier function of the epidermis.[25] Poor epidermal barrier function leads to increased transepidermal water loss, decreased skin hydration, and vulnerability to exogenous insults.[26] Skin barrier dysfunction might also be acquired secondary to irritants and mechanical disruption.[27] Damaged keratinocytes from the disrupted epidermal barrier may then trigger the recruitment and/or expansion of inflammatory cells via release of thymic stromal lymphopoietin and other cytokines.[28,29] Epidermal barrier breakdown also permits allergen penetration and binding to Langerhans cells, resulting in increased Th2 inflammation in the skin and systemically; this may also predispose toward atopic diseases, for example, asthma and food allergy.[22,23]

Inside-Out Hypothesis

The "inside-out" hypothesis posits that inflammation precedes and even causes barrier dysfunction in AD. Recent studies identified multiple polymorphisms of inflammatory genes in patients with AD, including IL-4 receptor-α (IL4Rα), IL-4, IL-13, IL-31, cluster of differentiation 14 (CD14), serine peptidase inhibitor, Kazal type 5, chemokine (C-C motif) ligand 5 (RANTES).[23,30–33] These polymorphisms may lead to (a) immune dysregulation and cutaneous inflammation, resulting in (b) impaired keratinocyte differentiation and function, followed by (c) downregulation of filaggrin and antimicrobial peptides (AMPs), thereby (d) allowing penetration of exogenous allergens.[23,25]

In summary, the outside-in and inside-out hypotheses differ on the sequence of events leading to disease manifestation. It may be that the outside-in hypothesis applies to a subset of patients, such as those with FLG polymorphisms, whereas the inside-out hypothesis applies in patients with polymorphisms of immune-related genes.[23] Regardless of "the chicken or the egg," both hypotheses agree that all patients have a combination of immune dysregulation, inflammation, and skin-barrier dysfunction.

ROLE OF INTERLEUKIN 4 AND INTERLEUKIN 13 IN ATOPIC DERMATITIS
Interleukin 4 and Interleukin 13 Activity in Atopic Dermatitis

IL-4 and IL-13 play prominent roles in inflammation, epidermal barrier dysfunction, itch, and susceptibility to infection in AD. In 1994, Hamid and colleagues[34] quantified IL-4 messenger RNA in skin biopsies of both acute and chronic lesions and nonlesional skin in AD patients and normal control skin. IL-4 gene expression was highest in acute AD lesions, but also increased in chronic AD lesions compared with nonlesional AD and normal control skin.[34] In 2001, transgenic murine models expressing epidermal IL-4 produced an AD-like phenotype, including pruritus, xerosis, inflammatory skin lesions, Staphylococcus aureus infection, and histopathology of chronic dermatitis with T cells, eosinophil infiltration, and elevation of total serum immunoglobulin (Ig) E and IgG1.[35] Other studies in both mice and humans substantiated the findings that IL-4 is increased in AD and that it may play a central role in pathogenesis.[36]

IL-13 has also been established as a critical cytokine in AD. Some studies have suggested that IL-13 may even be of greater pathophysiologic importance in AD than IL-4.[37] Increased expression of IL-13 also occurs in acute and chronic AD lesions in human skin, and transgenic mice with cutaneous IL-13 expression also develop an AD-like phenotype.[37–39] IL-13 is produced by multiple immune cells, including CD4+ and CD8+ T cells in AD lesions[40] as well as mast cells,[41] basophils,[42] and eosinophils.[43] Elevated IL-13 levels in AD lesions may initiate cutaneous inflammation and fibrotic remodeling.[44]

Interleukin 4, Interleukin 13, and Barrier Disruption in Atopic Dermatitis

As reviewed above, epidermal barrier dysfunction and keratinocyte damage are critical to the pathogenesis of AD (**Fig. 1**). Howell and colleagues[45] found that IL-4 and IL-13 inhibited filaggrin production in vitro during keratinocyte differentiation, suggesting that Th2 inflammation can result in acquired filaggrin deficiency and worsen barrier dysfunction overall. IL-4 and IL-13 were also found to downregulate keratinocyte expression of loricrin and involucrin, 2 important proteins for skin barrier formation and integrity.[46] Exposure to IL-4 in vitro was also found to reduce levels of ceramides, a class of important hydrophobic molecules in the stratum corneum, and desmoglein-3, a key protein in desmosomes.[47,48] In murine models, IL-4 has an inhibitory effect on barrier recovery, possibly by interfering with IL-1α effects, including DNA and lipid synthesis in keratinocytes.[49]

Interleukin 4, Interleukin 13, Immunoglobulin E, and Allergic Disease

IgE is central to allergic diseases, such as asthma, hay fever, and food allergy. IgE is produced by plasma cells upon stimulation with IL-4 and IL-13.[50] IgE binds to high-affinity receptors on

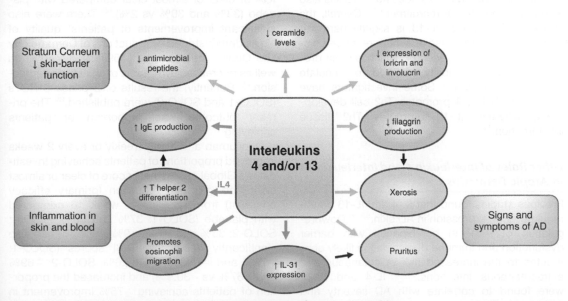

Fig. 1. Role of interleukins 4 and 13 in the pathogenesis of atopic dermatitis.

mast cells and basophils and can trigger the release of inflammatory mediators leading to type 1 mediated hypersensitivity reactions in allergic disease.[51] Patients with AD have significantly higher rates of asthma, hay fever, food allergy, and other allergic disorders.[1] Thus, many previously thought that IgE played a critical role in the pathophysiology of AD.[52] However, 20% to 50% of patients with AD may have normal total and allergen-specific IgE levels,[28] suggesting that IgE is not pathogenic in many AD patients. More recent paradigms have placed greater emphasis on the upstream T cells and T helper 2 inflammation, including IL-4 and IL-13, rather than the IgE downstream.[25]

IL-4 and IL-13 also play a critical role in asthma. IL-4 triggers IgE isotype switching, promotes eosinophil migration, increases mucus secretion, induces vascular cell adhesion molecule 1 expression, and causes Th2 differentiation.[53] In murine models, monoclonal antibodies to IL-4 before aerosol challenge neutralized Th2 inflammation that is integral for asthma pathogenesis.[54] Similarly, in murine models, selective blockade of IL-13 followed by antigen challenge failed to produce airway hyperresponsiveness, indicating that IL-13 is necessary for allergic asthma.[55] IL-13 has also been found to promote airway eosinophilia, activate macrophages, and increase airway mucus production.[56]

There is significant overlap in cytokine function as receptors for both IL-4 and IL-13 use the IL4Rα chain for signal transduction, but there are key differences. Both cytokines stimulate plasma cell IgE production, but IL-4 promotes Th2 cell differentiation, whereas IL-13 does not.[57] IL-4 is also involved in eosinophil recruitment.[36] Overall, the scope of function of IL-13 is slightly narrower than that of IL-4 because of a more restricted distribution of the IL-13 receptor, which is most pronounced by the inability of IL-13 to stimulate T-cell differentiation.[57] Some investigators have suggested that IL-4 promotes Th2 cell development, whereas IL-13 promotes Th2 tissue inflammation.[58]

Other Roles of Interleukin 4 and Interleukin 13 in Atopic Dermatitis

Previous studies found that IL-4 and IL-13 downregulate AMP expression in AD skin.[59,60] Downregulation of AMP in combination with barrier dysfunction and immune dysregulation likely contributes to the increased risk of cutaneous and extracutaneous infections.[61,62] IL-4 and IL-13 were found to correlate with AD severity and IL-31 levels.[63] Moreover, IL-4 was found to induce IL-31 expression by Th2 cells.[64] IL-31 appears to be an important inflammatory mediator of itch in AD.[65]

INTERLEUKIN 4 AND INTERLEUKIN 13 AS THERAPEUTIC TARGETS FOR ATOPIC DERMATITIS

With improved understanding of AD pathophysiology, IL-4 and IL-13 pathways have emerged as candidates for targeted therapy. There are several biologics targeting IL-4 and/or IL-13 pathways in development. The agent that is farthest along in the pipeline is dupilumab, a fully humanized monoclonal antibody targeting IL4Rα. IL4Rα is a subunit of the receptors for both IL-4 and IL-13.[66] Multiple early phase studies (I and IIa) of dupilumab for moderate to severe AD were published and showed significant improvement in various primary and secondary outcomes, including the Eczema Area and Severity Index (EASI), SCORing Atopic Dermatitis (SCORAD), body surface area (BSA) involvement, investigators global assessment (IGA), and numerical ratings scale (NRS)-itch.[67] In the phase 2b double-blind randomized controlled trial (RCT) (n = 379), dupilumab achieved significant improvement at 16 weeks in the EASI score (primary efficacy endpoint) at all doses, with maximum efficacy occurring at 300 mg weekly (−74%) or every 2 weeks (−68%) compared with placebo (−18%).[68] These doses also showed significant reductions of the SCORAD (−57% and −51%), BSA (−66% and −52%), and NRS-itch (−47% and −40%), with increased proportions of patients achieving an IGA of clear or almost clear compared with placebo (33% and 30% vs 2%).[68] There were also significant improvements of patients' quality of life as demonstrated by reductions of Dermatology Life Quality Index scores (−59% and −40%) as well as decreased symptoms of anxiety or depression.[69] Recently, the results of 2 phase 3 RCTs (SOLO-1 and SOLO-2) were published.[69] The primary outcome was proportion of patients achieving.

Dupilumab at 300 mg weekly or every 2 weeks improved proportions of patients achieving Investigator's Global Assessment score of clear or almost clear and ≥2-point reduction (primary efficacy endpoint) from baseline at week 16 compared with placebo (SOLO-1: 37% and 38% vs 10%; SOLO-2: 36% and 36% vs 9%).[69] Dupilumab also significantly decreased EASI scores (SOLO-1: −72% and −72.3% vs −37.6%; SOLO-2: −69% and −67% vs −30.9%) and increased the proportion of patients achieving ≥75% improvement in EASI (EASI-75) (SOLO-1: 53% and 51% vs 15%;

SOLO-2: 48% and 44% vs 12%). Dupilumab also improved several other clinical endpoints, including pruritus, symptoms of anxiety/depression, and quality of life. Interestingly, dupilumab was associated with lower rates of bacterial skin infections than placebo in early phase studies.[67–69] Across all the trials, dupilumab demonstrated very good safety with mainly mild or moderate adverse events. Injection site reactions (8%–19% vs 6%) and conjunctivitis of unclear cause (3%–5% vs $\leq$1%) were increased in patients treated with dupilumab compared with placebo.

Other agents targeting IL-13 pathways are in the pipeline for AD. Lebrikizumab is a monoclonal antibody that binds to IL-13. A phase 2 RCT to evaluate the safety and efficacy of lebrikizumab in patients with persistent moderate to severe AD that was inadequately controlled by TCS was performed. Lebrikizumab 125-mg injections every 4 weeks combined with twice daily midpotency TCS improved the proportion of patients achieving an EASI-50 at 12 weeks (primary efficacy endpoint) compared with placebo and TCS (82.4% vs 62.3%).[69] Lebrikizumab every 4 weeks also significantly improved the proportion of patients achieving an EASI-75 and EASI-90, but showed nonsignificant improvement in the IGA.[70] Larger-scale and later-phase studies are needed to confirm these findings and optimize potential dosing regimen.

Tralokinumab, an anti-IL-13 monoclonal antibody, may also be an effective therapy for AD. A phase 2b RCT was performed to evaluate the safety and efficacy of tralokinumab, another promising anti-IL13 monoclonal antibody, in adults age 18 years or older with moderate-severe AD. Tralokinumab 300mg subcutaneous compared with placebo injections every 2 weeks combined with mid-potency topical corticosteroids significantly reduced EASI, SCORAD, DLQI, and NRS-itch scores, and significantly increased the proportion of patients achieving and EASI50 and EASI75 at 12 weeks.[71] These biologics targeting Th2 inflammation are part of a novel treatment class that appears to be safe and effective for the management AD. There is some ongoing controversy about whether IL-4 or IL-13 plays a more important role in AD. The demonstrated efficacy of lebrikizumab and tralokinumab suggests that IL-13 may be a more important player than IL-4 and that IL-13 blockade may be sufficient for many patients with AD.

Agents targeting these pathways may also have utility in disorders such as asthma and chronic sinusitis with nasal polyposis. A clinical trial for dupilumab use in asthmatics with eosinophilia demonstrated fewer exacerbations and improved lung function.[72] Another trial showed efficacy of subcutaneous dupilumab for chronic sinusitis and nasal polyposis refractory to intranasal corticosteroids.[73] Lebrikizumab showed promising results in phase 2[74] and 3[75] studies of moderate to severe asthma. Tralokinumab has encountered mixed efficacy for asthma in clinical trials.[76,77]

SUMMARY

The current understanding of Th2 cytokine IL-4 and IL-13 involvement in AD pathophysiology has facilitated the development of novel biologics for AD. These novel agents are more targeted than the current systemic agents used off-label in the management of moderate to severe AD, with potentially better safety and efficacy. The age of biologics in AD has arrived!

REFERENCES

1. Silverberg JI, Simpson EL. Association between severe eczema in children and multiple comorbid conditions and increased healthcare utilization. Pediatr Allergy Immunol 2013;24(5):476–86.
2. Yu SH, Attarian H, Zee P, et al. Burden of sleep and fatigue in US adults with atopic dermatitis. Dermatitis 2016;27(2):50–8.
3. Silverberg JI, Garg NK, Paller AS, et al. Sleep disturbances in adults with eczema are associated with impaired overall health: a US population-based study. J Invest Dermatol 2015;135(1):56–66.
4. Garg N, Silverberg JI. Association between childhood allergic disease, psychological comorbidity, and injury requiring medical attention. Ann Allergy Asthma Immunol 2014;112(6):525–32.
5. Yu SH, Silverberg JI. Association between atopic dermatitis and depression in US adults. J Invest Dermatol 2015;135(12):3183–6.
6. Strom MA, Fishbein AB, Paller AS, et al. Association between atopic dermatitis and attention deficit hyperactivity disorder in U.S. children and adults. Br J Dermatol 2016;175(5):920–9.
7. Heinl D, Prinsen CA, Sach T, et al. Measurement properties of quality-of-life measurement instruments for infants, children and adolescents with eczema: a systematic review. Br J Dermatol 2016. [Epub ahead of print].
8. Kantor R, Dalal P, Cella D, et al. Research letter: impact of pruritus on quality of life: a systematic review. J Am Acad Dermatol 2016;75(5):885–6.e4.
9. Silverberg JI, Hanifin JM. Adult eczema prevalence and associations with asthma and other health and demographic factors: a US population-based study. J Allergy Clin Immunol 2013;132(5):1132–8.

10. Silverberg JI. Association between adult atopic dermatitis, cardiovascular disease, and increased heart attacks in three population-based studies. Allergy 2015;70(10):1300–8.

11. Silverberg JI, Silverberg NB, Lee-Wong M. Association between atopic dermatitis and obesity in adulthood. Br J Dermatol 2012;166(3):498–504.

12. Garg N, Silverberg JI. Association between eczema and increased fracture and bone or joint injury in adults: a US population-based study. JAMA Dermatol 2015;151(1):33–41.

13. Zhang A, Silverberg JI. Association of atopic dermatitis with being overweight and obese: a systematic review and metaanalysis. J Am Acad Dermatol 2015;72(4):606–16.e4.

14. Mohan GC, Silverberg JI. Association of vitiligo and alopecia areata with atopic dermatitis: a systematic review and meta-analysis. JAMA Dermatol 2015; 151(5):522–8.

15. Garg NK, Silverberg JI. Eczema is associated with osteoporosis and fractures in adults: a US population-based study. J Allergy Clin Immunol 2015;135(4):1085–7.e2.

16. Silverberg JI. Practice gaps in pruritus. Dermatol Clin 2016;34(3):257–61.

17. Silverberg JI, Nelson DB, Yosipovitch G. Addressing treatment challenges in atopic dermatitis with novel topical therapies. J Dermatolog Treat 2016;27(6): 568–76.

18. Zuberbier T, Orlow SJ, Paller AS, et al. Patient perspectives on the management of atopic dermatitis. J Allergy Clin Immunol 2006;118(1):226–32.

19. Eichenfield LF, Tom WL, Berger TG, et al. Guidelines of care for the management of atopic dermatitis: section 2. Management and treatment of atopic dermatitis with topical therapies. J Am Acad Dermatol 2014;71(1):116–32.

20. Roekevisch E, Spuls PI, Kuester D, et al. Efficacy and safety of systemic treatments for moderate-to-severe atopic dermatitis: a systematic review. J Allergy Clin Immunol 2014;133(2):429–38.

21. Yiu ZZ, Warren RB. Efficacy and safety of emerging immunotherapies in psoriasis. Immunotherapy 2015; 7(2):119–33.

22. Cork MJ, Robinson DA, Vasilopoulos Y, et al. New perspectives on epidermal barrier dysfunction in atopic dermatitis: gene-environment interactions. J Allergy Clin Immunol 2006;118(1):3–21 [quiz: 22–3].

23. Silverberg NB, Silverberg JI. Inside out or outside in: does atopic dermatitis disrupt barrier function or does disruption of barrier function trigger atopic dermatitis? Cutis 2015;96(6):359–61.

24. Palmer CN, Irvine AD, Terron-Kwiatkowski A, et al. Common loss-of-function variants of the epidermal barrier protein filaggrin are a major predisposing factor for atopic dermatitis. Nat Genet 2006;38(4): 441–6.

25. Malajian D, Guttman-Yassky E. New pathogenic and therapeutic paradigms in atopic dermatitis. Cytokine 2015;73(2):311–8.

26. Kabashima K. New concept of the pathogenesis of atopic dermatitis: interplay among the barrier, allergy, and pruritus as a trinity. J Dermatol Sci 2013;70(1):3–11.

27. Fluhr JW, Akengin A, Bornkessel A, et al. Additive impairment of the barrier function by mechanical irritation, occlusion and sodium lauryl sulphate in vivo. Br J Dermatol 2005;153(1):125–31.

28. Leung DY. New insights into atopic dermatitis: role of skin barrier and immune dysregulation. Allergol Int 2013;62(2):151–61.

29. Oyoshi MK, Larson RP, Ziegler SF, et al. Mechanical injury polarizes skin dendritic cells to elicit a T(H)2 response by inducing cutaneous thymic stromal lymphopoietin expression. J Allergy Clin Immunol 2010;126(5):976–84, 984.e1–5.

30. Hanifin JM. Evolving concepts of pathogenesis in atopic dermatitis and other eczemas. J Invest Dermatol 2009;129(2):320–2.

31. Novak N, Kruse S, Potreck J, et al. Single nucleotide polymorphisms of the IL18 gene are associated with atopic eczema. J Allergy Clin Immunol 2005;115(4): 828–33.

32. Oiso N, Fukai K, Ishii M. Interleukin 4 receptor alpha chain polymorphism Gln551Arg is associated with adult atopic dermatitis in Japan. Br J Dermatol 2000;142(5):1003–6.

33. Schulz F, Marenholz I, Folster-Holst R, et al. A common haplotype of the IL-31 gene influencing gene expression is associated with nonatopic eczema. J Allergy Clin Immunol 2007;120(5):1097–102.

34. Hamid Q, Boguniewicz M, Leung DY. Differential in situ cytokine gene expression in acute versus chronic atopic dermatitis. J Clin Invest 1994;94(2):870–6.

35. Chan LS, Robinson N, Xu L. Expression of interleukin-4 in the epidermis of transgenic mice results in a pruritic inflammatory skin disease: an experimental animal model to study atopic dermatitis. J Invest Dermatol 2001;117(4):977–83.

36. Brandt EB, Sivaprasad U. Th2 cytokines and atopic dermatitis. J Clin Cell Immunol 2011;2(3):110.

37. Tazawa T, Sugiura H, Sugiura Y, et al. Relative importance of IL-4 and IL-13 in lesional skin of atopic dermatitis. Arch Dermatol Res 2004;295(11):459–64.

38. Hamid Q, Naseer T, Minshall EM, et al. In vivo expression of IL-12 and IL-13 in atopic dermatitis. J Allergy Clin Immunol 1996;98(1):225–31.

39. Zheng T, Oh MH, Oh SY, et al. Transgenic expression of interleukin-13 in the skin induces a pruritic dermatitis and skin remodeling. J Invest Dermatol 2009;129(3):742–51.

40. Hijnen D, Knol EF, Gent YY, et al. CD8(+) T cells in the lesional skin of atopic dermatitis and psoriasis patients are an important source of IFN-gamma, IL-13, IL-17, and IL-22. J Invest Dermatol 2013;133(4):973–9.

41. Burd PR, Thompson WC, Max EE, et al. Activated mast cells produce interleukin 13. J Exp Med 1995;181(4):1373–80.

42. Li H, Sim TC, Alam R. IL-13 released by and localized in human basophils. J Immunol 1996;156(12):4833–8.

43. Schmid-Grendelmeier P, Altznauer F, Fischer B, et al. Eosinophils express functional IL-13 in eosinophilic inflammatory diseases. J Immunol 2002;169(2):1021–7.

44. Oh MH, Oh SY, Yu J, et al. IL-13 induces skin fibrosis in atopic dermatitis by thymic stromal lymphopoietin. J Immunol 2011;186(12):7232–42.

45. Howell MD, Kim BE, Gao P, et al. Cytokine modulation of atopic dermatitis filaggrin skin expression. J Allergy Clin Immunol 2007;120(1):150–5.

46. Kim BE, Leung DY, Boguniewicz M, et al. Loricrin and involucrin expression is down-regulated by Th2 cytokines through STAT-6. Clin Immunol 2008;126(3):332–7.

47. Hatano Y, Terashi H, Arakawa S, et al. Interleukin-4 suppresses the enhancement of ceramide synthesis and cutaneous permeability barrier functions induced by tumor necrosis factor-alpha and interferon-gamma in human epidermis. J Invest Dermatol 2005;124(4):786–92.

48. Kobayashi J, Inai T, Morita K, et al. Reciprocal regulation of permeability through a cultured keratinocyte sheet by IFN-gamma and IL-4. Cytokine 2004;28(4–5):186–9.

49. Kurahashi R, Hatano Y, Katagiri K. IL-4 suppresses the recovery of cutaneous permeability barrier functions in vivo. J Invest Dermatol 2008;128(5):1329–31.

50. Shirakawa I, Deichmann KA, Izuhara I, et al. Atopy and asthma: genetic variants of IL-4 and IL-13 signalling. Immunol Today 2000;21(2):60–4.

51. Gauchat JF, Henchoz S, Mazzei G, et al. Induction of human IgE synthesis in B cells by mast cells and basophils. Nature 1993;365(6444):340–3.

52. Fernandez-Benitez M. Etiologic implication of foods in atopic dermatitis: evidence in favor. Allergol Immunopathol (Madr) 2002;30(3):114–20 [in Spanish].

53. Steinke JW, Borish L. Th2 cytokines and asthma. Interleukin-4: its role in the pathogenesis of asthma, and targeting it for asthma treatment with interleukin-4 receptor antagonists. Respir Res 2001;2(2):66–70.

54. Corry DB, Folkesson HG, Warnock ML, et al. Interleukin 4, but not interleukin 5 or eosinophils, is required in a murine model of acute airway hyperreactivity. J Exp Med 1996;183(1):109–17.

55. Wills-Karp M, Luyimbazi J, Xu X, et al. Interleukin-13: central mediator of allergic asthma. Science 1998;282(5397):2258–61.

56. Ingram JL, Kraft M. IL-13 in asthma and allergic disease: asthma phenotypes and targeted therapies. J Allergy Clin Immunol 2012;130(4):829–42 [quiz: 843–4].

57. de Vries JE. The role of IL-13 and its receptor in allergy and inflammatory responses. J Allergy Clin Immunol 1998;102(2):165–9.

58. Sehra S, Yao Y, Howell MD, et al. IL-4 regulates skin homeostasis and the predisposition toward allergic skin inflammation. J Immunol 2010;184(6):3186–90.

59. Nomura I, Goleva E, Howell MD, et al. Cytokine milieu of atopic dermatitis, as compared to psoriasis, skin prevents induction of innate immune response genes. J Immunol 2003;171(6):3262–9.

60. Ong PY, Ohtake T, Brandt C, et al. Endogenous antimicrobial peptides and skin infections in atopic dermatitis. N Engl J Med 2002;347(15):1151–60.

61. Silverberg JI, Silverberg NB. Childhood atopic dermatitis and warts are associated with increased risk of infection: a US population-based study. J Allergy Clin Immunol 2014;133(4):1041–7.

62. Strom MA, Silverberg JI. Association between atopic dermatitis and extracutaneous infections in US adults. Br J Dermatol 2017;176(2):495–7.

63. Raap U, Weissmantel S, Gehring M, et al. IL-31 significantly correlates with disease activity and Th2 cytokine levels in children with atopic dermatitis. Pediatr Allergy Immunol 2012;23(3):285–8.

64. Stott B, Lavender P, Lehmann S, et al. Human IL-31 is induced by IL-4 and promotes TH2-driven inflammation. J Allergy Clin Immunol 2013;132(2):446–54.e5.

65. Sonkoly E, Muller A, Lauerma AI, et al. IL-31: a new link between T cells and pruritus in atopic skin inflammation. J Allergy Clin Immunol 2006;117(2):411–7.

66. Kotowicz K, Callard RE, Friedrich K, et al. Biological activity of IL-4 and IL-13 on human endothelial cells: functional evidence that both cytokines act through the same receptor. Int Immunol 1996;8(12):1915–25.

67. Beck LA, Thaci D, Hamilton JD, et al. Dupilumab treatment in adults with moderate-to-severe atopic dermatitis. N Engl J Med 2014;371(2):130–9.

68. Thaci D, Simpson EL, Beck LA, et al. Efficacy and safety of dupilumab in adults with moderate-to-severe atopic dermatitis inadequately controlled by topical treatments: a randomised, placebo-controlled, dose-ranging phase 2b trial. Lancet 2016;387(10013):40–52.

69. Simpson EL, Gadkari A, Worm M, et al. Dupilumab therapy provides clinically meaningful improvement in patient-reported outcomes (PROs): a phase IIb, randomized, placebo-controlled, clinical trial in adult patients with moderate to severe atopic dermatitis (AD). J Am Acad Dermatol 2016;75(3):506–15.

70. Efficacy and safety of lebrikizumab in patients with atopic dermatitis: a Phase II randomized, controlled trial (TREBLE) [press release]. European Academy of Dermatology and Venerology Annual Meeting. Vienna, Austria, October 1, 2016.

71. Wollenberg A, Howell MD, Guttman-Yassky E, et al. A phase 2b dose-ranging efficacy and safety study of tralokinumab in adult patients with moderate to severe atopic dermatitis (AD). Presented at the 75th Annual Meeting of the American Academy of Dermatology. Orlando, March 3–7, 2017.

72. Wenzel S, Ford L, Pearlman D, et al. Dupilumab in persistent asthma with elevated eosinophil levels. N Engl J Med 2013;368(26):2455–66.

73. Bachert C, Mannent L, Naclerio RM, et al. Effect of subcutaneous Dupilumab on nasal polyp burden in patients with chronic sinusitis and nasal polyposis: a randomized clinical trial. JAMA 2016;315(5): 469–79.

74. Hanania NA, Noonan M, Corren J, et al. Lebrikizumab in moderate-to-severe asthma: pooled data from two randomised placebo-controlled studies. Thorax 2015;70(8):748–56.

75. Hanania NA, Korenblat P, Chapman KR, et al. Efficacy and safety of lebrikizumab in patients with uncontrolled asthma (LAVOLTA I and LAVOLTA II): replicate, phase 3, randomised, double-blind, placebo-controlled trials. Lancet Respir Med 2016; 4(10):781–96.

76. Brightling CE, Chanez P, Leigh R, et al. Efficacy and safety of tralokinumab in patients with severe uncontrolled asthma: a randomised, double-blind, placebo-controlled, phase 2b trial. Lancet Respir Med 2015;3(9):692–701.

77. Piper E, Brightling C, Niven R, et al. A phase II placebo-controlled study of tralokinumab in moderate-to-severe asthma. Eur Respir J 2013; 41(2):330–8.

Long-Term Treatment of Atopic Dermatitis

James C. Prezzano, MD*, Lisa A. Beck, MD

KEYWORDS

- Long-term • Atopic dermatitis • Eczema • Treatment • Topical therapy • Systemic therapy

KEY POINTS

- Proactive, twice weekly therapy with either a topical corticosteroid or topical calcineurin inhibitor can decrease frequency of flares in patients with moderate to severe disease.
- The long-term efficacy and safety of current systemic treatments for atopic dermatitis is poorly studied and comparative trials are low powered; newer, safer alternatives are needed.
- Cyclosporine is the second-line agent with the most evidence of efficacy, and phototherapy is likely the safest.
- Methotrexate or mycophenolate mofetil/sodium may be as efficacious as cyclosporine for long-term use with potentially fewer side effects.
- Additional evidence is required before a definitive recommendation can be made.

INTRODUCTION

Atopic dermatitis (AD) is a common inflammatory systemic disease characterized by eczematous skin lesions and pruritus, and frequently accompanied by a host of other allergic disorders that manifest in the upper or lower airways, eyes, and/or the gastrointestinal tract. Therefore, the ideal, long-term management of AD may need to address both the cutaneous and systemic inflammation that is present in the circulation and even in distant organs. There is little consensus on what constitutes "long-term" treatment for chronic, inflammatory diseases. For example, in rheumatoid arthritis, long-term treatment has been defined as 1 year or longer.[1] In contrast, 12 weeks has been referred to as "long-term" in AD literature, which may simply reflect the paucity of interventional randomized, controlled trials (RCTs) greater than 3 months in duration.[2]

Outcome measures in the trials vary widely, making direct comparisons between trials and consequently between treatments or treatment regimens difficult. This literature uses terms such as remission, relapse, flare, and rebound, but how these terms are defined is not always clear or consistent.[3] Fortunately, the Harmonizing Outcome Measures for Eczema group is working toward standardizing outcome measures so trial comparisons in the future may be more accurate and informative (**Box 1**).[4]

METHOD

RCTs of 12 weeks or longer were identified by a Pubmed search for terms "atopic dermatitis," "atopic eczema," and "long-term" along with a review of the Global Resource of Eczema Trials database (greatdatabase.org.uk), consensus papers, and systematic reviews.[5–7] Repeated short

Disclosure Statement: Regeneron Pharmaceuticals – Co-investigator (J.C. Prezzano). Regeneron Pharmaceuticals – Investigator and Consultant; AbbVie (GR503814), Array BioPharma, Celgene, Genentech, Ironwood, Janssen, Leo Pharma, Lilly, MedImmune, Novartis, Regeneron Pharmaceuticals (GR524525), Unilever and Ziarco – honoraria, advisory board, or consulting fees (L.A. Beck).
Department of Dermatology, University of Rochester Medical Center, 601 Elmwood Avenue, Rochester, NY 14642, USA
* Corresponding author. Box 697, 601 Elmwood Avenue, Rochester, NY 14642.
E-mail address: James_Prezzano@urmc.rochester.edu

Dermatol Clin 35 (2017) 335–349
http://dx.doi.org/10.1016/j.det.2017.02.007
0733-8635/17/© 2017 Elsevier Inc. All rights reserved.

Box 1
What is meant by an AD flare (relapse)?

- There is no consensus on the definition.
  - Thirty-five percent of trials in a recent review used an arbitrary cutoff (eg, Investigators Global Assessment >4).[3]
  - Twenty-three percent of trials used the need to step-up treatment, in the physicians or patients opinion.[3]
  - The remainder used a composite or had no relapse definition.[3]
  - Nonflared AD is referred to stabilized AD or in "remission."

Abbreviation: AD, atopic dermatitis.

courses of treatment were included as long as the cumulative treatment period was at least 12 weeks. Trials not searchable by Pubmed were excluded. Only trials with a primary outcome of treatment efficacy or safety were included. Trials were excluded if information deemed necessary were missing (eg, study population ages or duration of treatment).

BATHING

Bathing can hydrate the skin while promoting the removal of irritants and allergens.[6] Expert consensus recommends up to once daily bathing, for a short period of time with lukewarm water.[6] Application of a moisturizer or a topical antiinflammatory agent immediately after bathing, often referred to as the "soak and smear" technique, is strongly encouraged (**Box 2**).[6]

Cleanser composition and pH affect skin barrier structure and function.[6] Normal skin has a slightly acidic pH (pH 4–5.5).[6] Soap, which typically has an

Box 2
What is the literature[a] lacking?

- Optimal frequency or duration of bathing.
- Efficacy of the soak and smear technique.
- Optimal cleanser composition.
- Efficacy of bath additives (eg, oatmeal, Epsom salts, vinegar, or essential oils).
- Efficacy of water softeners.
- Comparison of soap versus synthetic detergents (Syndets).

[a] Long-term randomized, controlled trials in patients with atopic dermatitis.

alkaline pH, is thought to have detrimental effects on stratum corneum proteins and lipids.[6] Although there are no long-term RCTs evaluating cleansers, an acidic or neutral, nonsoap cleanser (eg, synthetic detergent [Syndet]) should be recommended to AD patients.[6]

Sodium Hypochlorite (Bleach) Baths and Antiseptics

Only 1 small, long-term RCT found that twice weekly bleach baths (along with 7 d/mo of intranasal mupirocin) had a significant reduction in eczema area and severity index (EASI) and body surface area (BSA) affected (**Table 1**). These pediatric patients were randomized after an episode of clinically infected AD treated with 2 weeks of oral cephalexin.[8] Compliance was similar between the groups. Surprisingly, bleach baths did not affect *Staphylococcus aureus* skin colonization as measured by standard culture techniques (**Box 3**).[8]

Box 3
What is the literature[a] lacking?

- Efficacy and safety of sodium hypochlorite (bleach) baths as a monotherapy.
- Relative efficacy of bleach baths in patients noncolonized versus patients with colonized/infected AD.
- When and how to use mupirocin or other topical or systemic antibacterials.
- Efficacy of antibacterial clothing (eg, silver-coated textiles).

[a] Long-term randomized, controlled trials in patients with atopic dermatitis.

MOISTURIZERS

Topical moisturizers contain variable amounts of emollient, occlusive, and humectant ingredients aimed at reversing the generalized xerosis and enhancing the barrier function measured by transepidermal water loss.[6]

One long-term trial found twice daily moisturization decreased the median time to relapse from 30 to more than 180 days compared with no moisturization.[26] In a long-term RCT in adults, moisturization with a 5% urea-based moisturizer decreased the risk of AD relapse by 37% versus a cream without urea (see **Table 1**).[9]

Several prescription emollient devices have received approval as medical devices: EpiCeram, Atopiclair, Mimyx, HylatopicPlus, Tetrix, Tropazone, Neosalus, Zenieva, Neosalus, and Eletone.

Table 1
Long-term randomized, controlled trials

	Randomized Controlled Trial	Investigational Agent	Control	Study Population (Age Range, Severity)	Duration of Treatment	No. of Subjects
Bleach	Huang et al,[8] 2009 (SB)	Intranasal mupirocin 7 d/mo plus sodium hypochlorite (bleach) baths 2×/wk	Intranasal petrolatum 7 d/mo plus plain water baths 2×/wk	6 mo–17 y moderate-severe	12 wk	31
Moisturizer	Åkerström et al,[9] 2015 (DB)	5% urea cream, Canoderm (ACO HUD Nordic, Sweden) BID	Miniderm without glycerol (ACO Hud Nordic, Upplands Väsby, Sweden) BID	≥18 y moderate on average	Until relapse or 26 wk	172
TCSs 2×/wk	Berth-Jones et al,[10] 2003 (DB)	Fluticasone propionate 0.05% cream or 0.005% ointment 2×/wk	Emollient base 2×/wk	12–65 y moderate-severe	16 wk	295
	Fukuie et al,[11] 2016 (SB)	Betamethasone valerate 0.12% (extremities) hydrocortisone butyrate 0.1% (face <2 y, trunk) or tacrolimus 0.03% (face for patients ≥2 y); 2×/wk	TCS during flares only (same treatments) BID	3 mo–7 y moderate-severe	52 wk	30
	Glazenburg et al,[12] 2009 (DB)	Fluticasone propionate 0.005% ointment 2×/wk	Vehicle 2×/wk	4–10 y moderate-severe	16 wk	75
	Hanifin et al,[13] 2002 (DB)	Fluticasone propionate 0.05% cream daily 4×/wk for 4 wk then 2×/wk for 16 wk	Vehicle daily 4×/wk for 4 wk then 2×/wk for 16 wk	3 mo–65 y moderate-severe	20 wk	231
	Jorizzo,[43] 1995 (SB)	Desonide 0.05% ointment BID	Hydrocortisone 1.0% ointment BID	<1–12 y mild-moderate	25 wk	36
	Kirkup et al,[14] 2003 (DB) (2 trials)	Fluticasone propionate 0.05% cream for flares BID	Hydrocortisone 1% cream or hydrocortisone butyrate 0.1% cream for flares BID	2–14 y moderate-severe	12 wk	265
	Luger et al,[15] 2004 (DB)	Triamcinolone acetonide 0.1% cream (trunk/limbs) and hydrocortisone acetonide cream 1% (face/neck, intertriginous area) for flares BID	Pimecrolimus 1% cream for flares BID	18–79 y moderate-severe	52 wk	658

(continued on next page)

Table 1
(continued)

Randomized Controlled Trial	Investigational Agent	Control	Study Population (Age Range, Severity)	Duration of Treatment	No. of Subjects
Mandelin et al,[16] 2010 (DB)	Hydrocortisone acetate 1% ointment (face/neck and intertriginous) and hydrocortisone butyrate 0.1% ointment for flares +7 d BID	Tacrolimus 0.1% ointment for AD flares + 7 d BID	≥18 y moderate-severe	52 wk	80
Peserico et al,[17] 2008 (DB)	Methylprednisolone aceponate 0.1% cream 2×/ wk plus emollient 5 d BID (and once daily on methylprednisolone days)	Emollient (Advabase; Intendis GmbH, Berlin, Germany) 7 d/wk BID	≥12 y moderate-severe	16 wk	221
Reitamo et al,[18] 2005 (DB)	Hydrocortisone butyrate 0.1% ointment (body) and hydrocortisone acetate 1% ointment (face/neck, intertriginous) for flares BID	Tacrolimus 0.1% ointment for flares BID	≥18 y moderate-severe	26 wk	972
Sigurgeirsson et al,[19] 2015	Low-mid potency TCS, selected by the investigator	Pimecrolimus 1% cream for flares	3–12 mo mild-moderate	260 wk	2418
Thomas,[44] 2002 (DB)	Hydrocortisone 1% ointment "when required" for 7 d, BID	Betamethasone valerate 0.1% ointment (3 d) and emollient (4 d) "when required" BID	1–15 y mild-moderate	18 wk	207

TCIs 2×/wk

Reference	Treatment	Comparator	Population/severity	Length	No.
Fukuie et al,[11] 2016 (SB)	See TCS				
Gollick et al,[20] 2008 (DB)	Pimecrolimus 1% cream for flares BID	Vehicle for flares BID	≥18 y mild-moderate	26 wk	543
Hanifin et al,[21] 2001 (DB)	Tacrolimus 0.1% or tacrolimus 0.03% ointment for flares BID	Vehicle for flares BID	16–79 y moderate-severe	12 wk	631
Soter et al,[22] 2001 (DB) (2 trials)					
Kapp,[45] 2002 (DB)	Pimecrolimus 1% cream for flares BID	Vehicle for flares BID	3–23 mo mild-severe	52 wk	250
Luger et al,[15] 2004 (DB)	See TCS				
Mandelin et al,[16] 2010 (DB)	See TCS				
Meurer,[46] 2002 (DB)	Pimecrolimus 1% cream for flares BID	Vehicle for flares BID	≥18 y moderate-severe/ moderate	24 wk	192/130
Meurer et al,[23] 2004 (DB)	Tacrolimus 0.1% or tacrolimus 0.03% ointment for flares BID	Vehicle for flares BID	2–15 y moderate-severe	12 wk	351
Paller,[47] 2001 (DB)					
Paller,[48] 2008 (DB)	Tacrolimus 0.03% 3×/wk/ tacrolimus 0.03% (2–15 y) or 0.1% (≥16 y) ointment 3×/wk	Vehicle 3×/wk	2–15 y moderate-severe/2–15 and ≥16 y	40 wk	105/197
Breneman et al,[49] 2008 (DB)					
Ruer-Mulard,[50] 2009 (DB)	Pimecrolimus 1% cream BID	Pimecrolimus 1% cream daily	2–17 y mild-severe	16 wk	268
Siegfried,[51] 2006 (DB)	Pimecrolimus 1% cream for flares BID	Vehicle for flares BID	3–143 mo mild-severe	24 wk	275
Sigurgeirsson,[52] 2008 (DB)	Pimecrolimus 1% cream for flares BID	Vehicle for flares BID	1–17 y mild-moderate	26 wk	521
Thaçi et al,[24] 2008 (DB)	Tacrolimus 0.03% ointment 2×/wk	Vehicle 2×/wk	2–15 y mild-severe/ moderate-severe	52 wk	250/153
Thaci et al,[53] 2010 (DB)	Pimecrolimus 1% for flares BID	Vehicle for flares BID	1–17 y mild-severe	52 wk	711
Wahn,[54] 2002 (DB)					
Wollenberg et al,[25] 2008 (DB)	Tacrolimus 0.1% 2×/wk	Vehicle 2×/wk	≥16 y mild-severe	52 wk	224

Length is of the controlled treatment period (or proactive/maintenance period), number of subjects is the number randomized to the ≥12-week period.

Patients receiving 2-3× per week treatment are proactive treatment with AD in remission. "Flares" is used interchangeably with first signs of AD. AD severity is as stated in trial.

Abbreviations: AD, atopic dermatitis; BID, twice daily; DB, double-blind; SB, single-blind; TCI, topical calcineurin inhibitors; TCS, topical corticosteroids.

The FDA 510(k) approval process is a less rigorous process than the standard premarket approval process most drugs go through.[6] Prescription emollient devices have ingredients thought to have skin hydration, antiinflammatory, or antipruritic properties. Unfortunately, there have been no long-term RCTs comparing these prescription creams with over-the-counter alternatives, some of which have also been formulated to replete AD deficiencies (eg, ceramides and filaggrin breakdown products).[6]

Expert consensus recommends frequent moisturizer use, ideally with a moisturizer that is free of additives, fragrances, perfumes, and other potential sensitizing agents.[6] Specific recommendations should be tailored to the extent and severity of AD, and based on physician and patient preference.[6,9] Petrolatum-based ointments are widely seen as effective and often do not contain potentially irritating preservatives.[6] Creams are a good alternative for AD patients who cannot tolerate ointments. Lotions should be avoided because they can cause a drying effect (**Box 4**).[6]

Box 4
What is the literature[a] lacking?

- More head-to-head trials with moisturizers.
- Ideal moisturizer formulation.
- Prescription emollient devices and over-the-counter moisturizers with filaggrin breakdown products and/or ceramides.
- Frequency of moisturization.

[a] Long-term randomized, controlled trials in patients with atopic dermatitis.

TOPICAL ANTIINFLAMMATORIES

The long-term topical antiinflammatory literature has examined both "reactive" treatment, that is, at the first signs and symptoms of an AD flare until resolved, and "proactive" treatment, that is, 2 to 3 weeks of treatment for nonflared AD (**Box 5**; see **Table 1**).

TOPICAL CORTICOSTEROIDS

Topical corticosteroids (TCS) assert broad, nonspecific antiinflammatory effects on a multitude of cell types, many of which are dysregulated in AD.[6] TCS are classified from mild (group I in Europe, class VII in the United States) to superpotent (group IV in Europe, class I in the United States) based on results from vasoconstriction assays.[6] There have been at least 110 TCS RCTs

---

Box 5
"Stabilized" atopic dermatitis

Most trials investigating the proactive use of topical antiinflammatories recruit patients who are flaring and treat until they reach a specific eczema score (ie, 50% improvement) and at this point they are considered "stabilized" or in remission. The patients are then randomized to either *proactive* or vehicle control to the site of previous atopic dermatitis lesions.

---

performed in patients with AD, with the results consistently demonstrating efficacy for the treatment of both active lesions and as prevention of flares (eg, proactive treatment).[5,6] Most of the trials were short in duration and of poor quality by today's data reporting standards.[5,6]

Long-Term Reactive Topical Corticosteroids Treatment Trials

RCTs have demonstrated safety and continued efficacy of repeated courses of low- to mid-potency TCS on active AD skin until clearance for up to 5 years in children and up to 1 year in adults.[15,16,19] Mid-potency TCS have been shown to be superior in efficacy over lower potency TCS for long-term reactive treatment in children (see **Table 1**).[14] The longest TCS RCT to date, enrolling patients in infancy, showed continued improvement in BSA affected and disease control (Investigators Global Assessment of 0 or 1) over the 5-year trial period using low- to mid-potency TCS.[19] This study argues against the notion that TCS lose effectiveness over time (tachyphylaxis).

Long-Term Proactive Topical Corticosteroids Prevention Trials

The proactive approach of applying low-mid potency TCS twice weekly (consecutive days or Thursday and Sunday) for the prevention of flares in stabilized AD has been shown to be effective in both adults and children (**Table 2**).[10,12,13,17]

Proactive treatment (along with reactive) was found to be superior to reactive only management in a yearlong RCT in pediatric patients.[11] Both groups showed improvements from baseline, but the proactive group was superior to the reactive group (Scoring Atopic Dermatitis [SCORAD] and quality of life scores).[11]

Long-Term Topical Corticosteroids Adverse Effects

When used properly, long-term use of low- to mid-potency TCS is well-tolerated. Potential adverse

Table 2
Reductions in relapse rate observed with proactive topical corticosteroids in moderate-severe atopic dermatitis

TCS	Pediatric	Adult	Trial
Fluticasone propionate 0.05% cream	5.1 times less likely	7.0 times less likely	Hanifen et al,[13] 2002
Fluticasone propionate 0.05% cream	5.8 times less likely[a]	5.8 times less likely[a]	Berth-Jones et al,[10] 2003
Methylprednisolone aceponate cream	3.5 times less likely[a]	3.5 times less likely[a]	Peserico et al,[17] 2008
Fluticasone propionate 0.005% ointment	2.18 times less likely (5.12 in females, 0.85 in males)	ND	Glazenburg et al,[12] 2009
Fluticasone propionate 0.005% ointment	1.9 times less likely[a]	1.9 times less likely[a]	Berth-Jones et al,[10] 2003

Abbreviation: ND, not done.
[a] Children aged ≥12 and adults, results not stratified.

effects (AEs) from their long-term use are rare but include atrophy, hypothalamic–pituitary–adrenal axis suppression and striae; the latter two have only been observed in RCTs with the use of mid-potency TCS used over a large BSA for months.[13,15,16,21] The use of twice weekly proactive treatment has not been shown to cause skin atrophy.[10–13,17]

Topical Corticosteroids Summary

TCS are first-line treatment for AD patients who have failed good skin care, including moisturizer use. For mild disease, the reactive approach of applying TCS at the first signs and symptoms of an AD flare is typically very effective. In patients with frequent relapses, the evidence supports an additional proactive approach, with intermittent use of low- to mid-potency TCS (**Box 6**). The optimal frequency for reactive treatment remains controversial, with some recently approved TCS recommended for once daily use (methylprednisolone aceponate, mometasone, or fluticasone).[5,6,10,17]

Box 6
What is the literature[a] for topical corticosteroids use?

- Randomized, controlled trials evaluating intermittent topical corticosteroids of greater than moderate potency.
- The effect of application frequency on disease resolution or relapse prevention.

[a] Long-term randomized, controlled trials in patients with atopic dermatitis.

TOPICAL CALCINEURIN INHIBITORS

TCIs are natural products of the fungus-like bacteria, *Streptomyces*, that inhibit calcineurin-dependent T-cell activation and block the production of proinflammatory cytokines (**Box 7**).[6] There are two available TCIs, tacrolimus ointment and pimecrolimus cream.

Long-Term Reactive Topical Calcineurin Inhibitor Treatment Trials

RCTs have demonstrated that TCIs are safe and effective when used twice daily for the intermittent treatment of AD flares in children and infants (≥3 months) for up to 5 years, and in adults for up to 1 year.[16,19] Statistically significant improvements were noted in EASI, Physicians Global Assessment, SCORAD, and BSA in infants (≥3 months), children, and adults (see **Table 1**).[16,19–23]

Long-Term Proactive Topical Calcineurin Inhibitor Trials

The proactive use of tacrolimus has been shown to be effective and safe for up to 1 year in both children (2–15 years, 0.03%) and adults (≥16 years, 0.1%; see **Table 1**).[24,25] A proactive

Box 7
Topical calcineurin inhibitors are approved for the following ages in the United States

- Pimecrolimus 1% cream: ≥2 years
- Tacrolimus 0.3% ointment: ≥2 years
- Tacrolimus 0.1% ointment: ≥16 years

approach prevents and delays AD flares compared with vehicle.[25]

Long-Term Topical Calcineurin Inhibitor Adverse Events

TCIs are considered very safe with most AEs reported as transient, mild, and at similar rates to the control or vehicle.[2] The most common AE is skin burning, which resolves in 80% of patients after 1 week.[22] Although some trials have found increased rates of minor infections (bronchitis, impetigo, nasopharyngitis, or infected eczema), the rates were low and no differences were seen in serious infections or AEs.[19] Since 2006, TCIs have had a boxed warning based on a theoretic risk of malignancy.[2,19] The largest and longest trial looking at infants treated with pimecrolimus found no evidence of increased malignancy risk, nor has a recent systematic review.[2,19]

Topical Calcineurin Inhibitor Summary

TCIs are a safe and effective treatment for both proactive and reactive long-term management of mild to moderate AD in infants through adults. TCIs provide an alternative to TCS and have no risk of hypothalamic–pituitary–adrenal axis alteration or striae; unfortunately, TCIs are only approved for patients 2 years or older, despite robust efficacy and favorable safety data in infants.[2,6,18,19]

COMPARISON TRIALS OF TOPICAL CORTICOSTEROIDS AND TOPICAL CALCINEURIN INHIBITORS

Two long-term RCTs in adults have demonstrated that tacrolimus 0.1% is more effective than hydrocortisone butyrate 0.1% ointment (class V) for the body and hydrocortisone acetate 1% (class VII) cream for the face.[16,18] Whereas mid-potency triamcinolone 0.1% cream (class IV) was slightly more effective than pimecrolimus to treat adult AD flares.[15] The PETITE trial (Five-Year Safety Study of Pimecrolimus Cream 1% in Infants 3 to Less Than 12 Months of Age With Mild to Moderate Atopic Dermatitis), which was the longest (5 years) RCT trial comparing reactive treatment with a TCI (pimecrolimus) to low- to mid-potency TCS in infants in children, found that both treatment options were safe and effective (see **Table 1**).[19] By the fifth year, more than 85% of patients (pimecrolimus 88.7%; TCS, 92.3%) achieved an Investigators Global Assessment of 1 or less (significance of differences not stated).[19] Not surprisingly, pimecrolimus was steroid sparing, with a median of only 7 days of

TCS rescue use (over 5 years) compared with 178 days in the TCS group.[19]

Topical Antiinflammatory Summary

Based on US Food and Drug Administration labeling, TCS are indicated as first-line therapy and TCIs are second-line therapy for AD. Despite this, studies have shown that both TCIs and TCS (low- to mid-potency) are generally safe and effective for long-term reactive and proactive use in patients with frequent flares. TCI use is a steroid-sparing strategy and eliminates some of the concerns associated with chronic TCS use. TCI use is limited by difficulty prescribing for infants, reduced efficacy compared with TCS, and burning with initial application (**Box 8**).

Box 8
What is the literature[a] lacking?

- RCTs investigating the use of both TCIs and TCS on the same site.
- Comparison trials with the proactive use of TCIs versus TCS.

Abbreviations: RCT, randomized, controlled trial; TCIs, topical calcineurin inhibitors; TCS, topical corticosteroids.
[a] Long-term randomized, controlled trials in patients with atopic dermatitis.

SYSTEMIC MANAGEMENT
Systemic Glucocorticoids

Glucocorticoids are the only US Food and Drug Administration–approved systemic pharmaceutical therapy for the treatment of AD. Unfortunately, there are no long-term RCTs evaluating efficacy and safety of systemic glucocorticoids in AD (**Box 9**). Their use should be limited to short courses as a transition to a more sustainable treatment. The most recent American Academy of Dermatology guidelines recommend an initial dose of 0.5 mg/kg/d followed by a slow taper to decrease the risk of rebound.[7] There is no consensus on the duration of the taper, but it should overlap with a steroid-sparing agent. Special consideration should be made with pediatric patients because of concerns with delayed or reduced bone growth.[7]

Long-Term Systemic Glucocorticoid Adverse Events

Rheumatoid arthritis literature has demonstrated that long-term treatment with even low-dose

---

Box 9
Long-term glucocorticoid[a] risk

- ≤5 mg: low risk[b]
- >5 to ≤10 mg: medium risk
- >10 mg: high risk

[a] Prednisone equivalent.
[b] Unless they are at high risk of cardiovascular disease.
From Patrizi A, Raone B, Ravaioli GM. Management of atopic dermatitis: safety and efficacy of phototherapy. Clin Cosmet Investig Dermatol 2015;8:511–20.

---

corticosteroids (≤15 mg/d prednisone equivalent) has serious side effects, including fractures, infections, gastrointestinal hemorrhage, and cataracts.[1] Prophylaxis against gastrointestinal hemorrhage and bone loss is encouraged for long-term use. The long-term AEs associated with intermittent pulse dosing of systemic glucocorticoids are poorly studied in AD.

PHOTOTHERAPY

Ultraviolet radiation is thought to improve AD by strengthening the barrier, modulating tissue inflammation, reducing pruritus and decreasing *S aureus* colonization (**Box 10**).[27] Although numerous types of phototherapy have been tried for AD, long-term RCTs have only investigated narrow band (NB) ultraviolet B (UVB) light, broadband ultraviolet A (UVA) light, UVA plus UVB (UVAB), and visible light phototherapy (**Table 3**).

Long-Term Phototherapy Randomized, Controlled Trials

A 12-week, double-blind RCT comparing biweekly NB-UVB, UVA, and visible light phototherapy in adolescents and adults found NB-UVB to be superior with greater reductions in disease activity (Six Area, Six Sign Atopic Dermatitis [SASSAD]) and extent (BSA) compared with visible light, and a greater reduction in extent compared with UVA.[29] No differences were observed between UVA and visible light.[29] In a yearlong RCT comparing UVAB and cyclosporine (CsA) treatment in adults, both treatments led to significant improvements in SCORAD, but CsA-treated patients improved faster and had significantly more days in remission than the UVAB group.[28] Additionally there were twice as many withdrawals in the UVAB group, mostly attributable to treatment failure.[28] Although more patients reported AEs in the CsA group, more patients withdrew because of AEs in the phototherapy group.

Long-Term Phototherapy Adverse Events

Phototherapy is generally well-tolerated, although the long-term risks vary by modality. Photodamage is a greater concern with UVA exposure.[27] Carcinogenesis, especially nonmelanomatous skin cancer, is the most feared concern and has been well-documented in UVA-based phototherapy with less known about the relative risk after NB-UVB treatment.[27]

Summary

Phototherapy, especially NB-UVB (which is more widely available), is a reasonable second-line treatment option for long-term management of moderate to severe AD. Larger studies are warranted to fully understand the ability of NB-UVB to induce disease remission and delay relapse (**Box 11**).

Box 10
Phototherapy options worldwide

- UVA (broadband): 315–400 nm
- UVA1: 340–400 nm
- UVB (broadband): 280–315 nm
- NB-UVB: 311 nm peak
- UVA and UVB (UVAB): 280–400 nm
- Visible light phototherapy: 400–700 nm

Abbreviations: NB-UVB, narrow band ultraviolet B light; UVA, ultraviolet A light; UVA1, ultraviolet A1 light; UVB, ultraviolet B light.

Box 11
What is the literature[a] lacking?

- Large cohort studies to determine the risk of photocarcinogenesis with newer therapies (NB-UVB and UVA1) and whether they are specific to AD patients.
- Risks and benefits of phototherapy combined with balneotherapy.
- Trials of phototherapy in children.

Abbreviations: AD, atopic dermatitis; NB-UVB, narrow band ultraviolet B light; UVA1, ultraviolet A1 light.
[a] Long-term randomized, controlled trials in patients with atopic dermatitis.

Table 3
Long-term systemic RCTs

	RCT	Investigational Agent	Control	Study Population (Age Range, Severity)	Duration of Treatment	No. of Subjects
Phototherapy	Granlund et al,[28] 2001	Intermittent UVAB[a] for 8-wk cycles	Intermittent CsA for 8-wk cycles, starting dose of 4 mg/kg/d	18–70 y severe	52 wk	72
	Reynolds et al,[29] 2001 (DB)	NB-UVB or Broadband UVA[a] 2×/wk	Visible light phototherapy 2×/wk	16–65 y moderate to severe	12 wk	73
CsA	Bemanian et al,[30] 2005	CsA 4 mg/kg/d	IVIG 2 g/kg (1 time)	Pediatric (mean 11.9 y and 6.4 y in CsA and IVIG), severe	12 wk	16
	El-Khalawany et al,[31] 2013	CsA 2.5 mg/kg/d	MTX 7.5 mg/wk	8–14 y severe	12 wk	40
	Granlund et al,[28] 2001	See phototherapy				
	Haeck et al,[32] 2011 (SB)	CsA 3 mg/kg/d	EC-MPS 1440 mg/d	≥18 y, severe	30 wk	50
	Harper et al,[33] 2000	Continuous CsA, starting/max dose 5 mg/kg/d, decreased based on response	12-wk courses of CsA, initial starting dose of 5 mg/kg/d, decreased on response, restarted at last dose	2–16 y severe	52 wk	40
	Koppelhus et al,[34] 2014 (crossover trial)	CsA 3 mg/kg/d	Extracorporeal photopheresis 2 consecutive days, 2×/mo	20–45 y severe	4 mo	20
	Zonneveld et al,[35] 1996	CsA starting dose 5 mg/kg/d and decreasing	CsA starting dose 3 mg/kg/d and increasing	18–70 y severe	≤52 wk	78
MTX	El-Khalawany et al,[31] 2013	See CsA				
	Schram et al,[36] 2011 (SB)	MTX (10–22 mg/wk)	AZA (1.5–2.5 mg/kg/d)	≥18 y (mean 40 y)	12 wk	42
EC-MPS	Haeck et al,[32] 2011 (SB)	See CsA				
AZA	Berth-Jones et al,[37] 2002 (DB) (crossover trial)	AZA 2.5 mg/kg/d	Placebo	17–73 y severe	12 wk	37
	Meggitt et al,[38] 2006 (DB)	AZA 2.5 mg/kg/d or 1 mg/kg/d based on TPMT activity	Placebo	16–65 y moderate to severe	12 wk	63
	Schram et al,[36] 2011 (SB)	See MTX				

Abbreviations: AZA, azathioprine; CsA, cyclosporine; DB, double blind; EC-MPS, enteric-coated mycophenolate sodium; IVIG, intravenous immunoglobulin; MTX, methotrexate; NB-UVB, narrow band ultraviolet A light; RCT, randomized, controlled trial; SB, single blind; TPMT, thiopurine methyltransferase; UVA, ultraviolet A light; UVB, ultraviolet B light.
[a] Limited availability.

CYCLOSPORINE

CsA is approved for the treatment of adults (ie, ≥16 years of age) with AD in at least 15 European countries, Australia, and Japan. CsA is an oral calcineurin inhibitor that suppresses the activation of the T-cell transcription factor, nuclear factor of activated T cells, inhibiting the transcription of a number of cytokines, including interleukin-2.[7,32] Generally, CsA has been viewed as a short-term or temporizing treatment for uncontrolled AD and used to transition (albeit more slowly than glucocorticoids) to a safer, longer term treatment. There is general consensus that continuous treatment with CSA beyond 1 to 2 years is not recommended.[7]

Long-Term Cyclosporine Randomized, Controlled Trials

CsA has been shown to be effective and relatively safe in 4 long-term RCTs in adults who received up to 1 year of continuous treatment (see **Table 3**).[28,32,34,35] Low starting doses (3 mg/kg/d) and high starting doses (5 mg/kg/d) were found to be equally effective (EASI/BSA improvement) after 2 weeks.[35] As mentioned, CsA was found to be superior to UVAB.[28] Lower dose CsA (3 mg/kg/d) was found to be equally effective to enteric coated-mycophenolate sodium (EC-MPS, 1440 mg/d) as a maintenance therapy for severe AD.[32] The EC-MPS group had a slower onset of action with 29% of the EC-MPS patients requiring short courses of systemic glucocorticoids compared with none in the CsA group.[32] In a small crossover RCT comparing 4 months of extracorporeal photopheresis with CsA (3 mg/kg/d), both treatments were equally effective for severe AD, although patients preferred extracorporeal photopheresis.[34]

CsA has been shown to be effective in 3 small RCTs in children (see **Table 3**).[30,31,33] Continuous CsA was compared with repeated 12-week courses of CsA (started at relapse/flare) in a yearlong RCT in children with severe AD.[33] Both groups had significant, sustained improvements in SASSAD, but continuous treatment provided more consistent control.[33] A 12-week RCT comparing CsA (2.5 mg/kg/d) with methotrexate (MTX, 7.5 mg/wk) found both drugs at these lower doses to be equally effective in reducing SCORAD.[31] Both drugs were well-tolerated with no AEs necessitating drug discontinuation or dose reduction.[31] In a very small 3-month pediatric trial, CsA (4 mg/kg/d) was found to be superior to intravenous immunoglobulin (2 g/kg once) as assessed by reduction in SCORAD with both being well-tolerated (**Box 12**).[30]

Long-Term Cyclosporine Adverse Events

Irreversible nephrotoxicity, hypertension, and nonmelanomatous skin cancer are the major, serious AEs. Kidney biopsies performed on psoriatic patients treated with CsA (2.5–6 mg/kg/d), found increasing evidence of nephropathy over time with all biopsies showing some pathology after 2 years of treatment, although biopsies showed only mild changes until more than 2 years of treatment.[39] Two or more months with serum creatinine more than 30% above baseline may predict irreversible nephrotoxicity.[40] The majority of side effects seen in the AD RCT literature were reversible and included hypertension and transient increases in serum creatinine.[28,33,35]

Summary

Based on 7 long-term RCTs, CsA can be recommended as an effective second line agent for AD for up to 1 to 2 years in both adults and children 2 years and older.[28,30–35] Larger long-term studies are needed to fully elucidate nephrotoxicity risk specific to AD patients. Long-term RCTs assessing weekend or intermittent dosing of CsA are recommended to further evaluate these potentially renal-sparing regimens.

Box 12
What is the literature lacking for cyclosporine?

- Nephrotoxicity risk in atopic dermatitis subpopulations (age, gender, race, and comorbidities)
- Dosing regimens that may reduce the risk of nephrotoxicity, including intermittent or weekend dosing.

METHOTREXATE

MTX is an antimetabolite that blocks synthesis of DNA, RNA, and purines and is thought to inhibit T-cell function.[7] The long-term studies with MTX for the treatment of AD are few, but promising.

Long-Term Methotrexate Randomized, Controlled Trials

In an RCT comparing MTX (10–22 mg/wk) with azathioprine (AZA, 1.5–2.5 mg/kg/d) in adults with severe AD, both treatments were found to have similar effects on disease severity (based on a number of assessment tools), including reductions in SCORAD of 42% versus 39% in MTX versus AZA, respectively.[36]

MTX (7.5 mg/wk) compared favorably with CsA (2.5 mg/kg/d) in children aged 8 to 14 years with SCORAD reductions of 49% (vs 45% in CsA, difference not significant) over 12 weeks.[31] The MTX group had a delayed onset of action of approximately 3 to 5 weeks versus 2 to 3 weeks in the CsA group, but a longer time to relapse after drug discontinuation (20 vs 14 weeks).[31]

Long-Term Methotrexate Adverse Events

The RCTs in AD suggest MTX is well-tolerated, although the currently available literature is underpowered (n = 42; n = 40) to find anything but the most common AEs, such as nausea.[7,31,36] The most serious long-term risks are pulmonary fibrosis and hepatotoxicity, but some authors have suggested that AD patients may be at lower risk than psoriasis patients owing to their reduced rates of obesity and alcoholism.[7]

Summary

Based on only 2 small long-term RCTs, MTX seems to be a well-tolerated and effective second- or third-line option for the long-term treatment of moderate-severe AD in both children (≥8 years) and adults (**Box 13**).[31,36]

> **Box 13**
> **What is the methotrexate literature[a] lacking?**
>
> - Larger and longer studies in children and adults.
> - Dose finding trials.
>
> [a] Long-term randomized, controlled trials in patients with atopic dermatitis.

AZATHIOPRINE

AZA works by inhibiting DNA production of high proliferation cells such as B and T lymphocytes.[7]

Long-Term Azathioprine Randomized Controlled Trials

Two adult RCTs have shown AZA to be more effective than placebo over 12 weeks.[37,38] SASSAD sign score decreased by 37% versus 20% in patients with moderate to severe AD treated with either 1 or 2.5 mg/kg/d based on thiopurine methyltransferase activity over placebo.[38] In a small crossover trial testing 2.5 mg/kg/d in severe AD, the treatment had a 26% SASSAD reduction compared with 3% in the placebo group.[37] In a comparative study with MTX in adults over 12 weeks, both treatments had similar SCORAD improvements from baseline (see MTX).[36]

Long-Term Azathioprine Adverse Events

AZA was not always well-tolerated, the AZA groups had high dropout rates (32%, 15%, 14%), and higher rates of serious AEs, including 2 of 42 patients developing potentially serious AZA hypersensitivity in 1 trial.[36–38] Side effects in the other RCTs included severe nausea and vomiting, headaches, and minor laboratory abnormalities.[37] Additionally, AZA has been linked to cutaneous and lymphoproliferative malignancies[7] (**Box 14**).

Summary

Although AZA has been shown to be modestly effective for long-term treatment in adults with AD, tolerability and AEs limit it to a third- or fourth-line option.

> **Box 14**
> **What is the azathioprine literature lacking?**
>
> - Larger and longer trials.

MYCOPHENOLIC ACID PRECURSORS

Mycophenolic acid prevents purine synthesis in B and T cells by inhibiting inosine monophosphate dehydrogenase.[32] Both mycophenolate mofetil and EC-MPS are prodrugs of mycophenolic acid. EC-MPS was formulated to decrease gastrointestinal AEs.[32] The only long-term RCT investigating EC-MPS showed similar efficacy of EC-MPS (1440 mg/d) to CsA (3 mg/kg/d) in adults after the 10th week of therapy, but a delayed onset of action in the EC-MPS group.[32] EC-MPS may represent a promising third-line agent, although larger long-term RCTs are required before a recommendation can be made.

EMERGING THERAPIES WITH PHASE III DATA
Crisaborole

Crisaborole is a topical phosphodiesterase-4 inhibitor that reduces the production of proinflammatory cytokines by slowing the degradation of cyclic adenosine monophosphate.[41] In 2 large (n = 759 and n = 763), double-blind RCTs in children (≥2 years of age) and adults with mild to moderate AD, crisaborole ointment significantly improved disease severity, with 32.8% of crisaborole-treated patients achieving a score of clear or almost clear versus 25.4% in the vehicle group after 29 days.[41] Long-term and comparative trials with other topical treatments are recommended for this potentially new class of therapy and to better assess long-term tolerability.

Dupilumab

Dupilumab is a fully human monoclonal antibody directed against the interleukin (IL)-4α receptor α-subunit, which blocks the signaling of both IL-4 and IL-13, the 2 key drivers of type 2 immune response. Two large (n = 671 and n = 708), long-term (16 weeks) double-blind RCTs evaluating adults with moderate to severe AD demonstrated that subcutaneous dupilumab was superior to placebo in all prespecified efficacy endpoints including clinical severity (EASI) and extent of involvement (BSA).[42] The overall incidence of AEs was similar to the placebo group, with most being mild to moderate.[42] Dupilumab seems to be a highly effective and safe systemic treatment for adults with moderate to severe AD.

SUMMARY

Long-term treatment for AD begins with optimization of skin care including frequent moisturizer use and graded, reactive topical antiinflammatory use. The addition of proactive TCI or low-mid potency TCS therapy at sites of frequent relapse represent the next step in treatment. There are a limited number of long-term RCTs evaluating the safety and/or efficacy of systemic treatments with the most robust data for CsA. EC-MPS or MTX may be as effective as CsA (mid-dose) with fewer safety concerns. Crisaborole and dupilumab are exciting new therapies with robust evidence of efficacy to mild to moderate and moderate to severe AD, respectively. Should they gain US Food and Drug Administration approval, they will markedly improve our armamentarium to address this chronic inflammatory skin disorder.

REFERENCES

1. Saag KG, Koehnke R, Caldwell JR, et al. Low dose long-term corticosteroid therapy in rheumatoid arthritis: an analysis of serious adverse events. Am J Med 1994;96:115–23.
2. Siegfried EC, Jaworski JC, Kaiser JD, et al. Systematic review of published trials: long-term safety of topical corticosteroids and topical calcineurin inhibitors in pediatric patients with atopic dermatitis. BMC Pediatr 2016;16:75.
3. Barbarot S, Rogers NK, Abuabara K, et al. Strategies used for measuring long-term control in atopic dermatitis trials: a systematic review. J Am Acad Dermatol 2016;75(5):1038–44.
4. Schmitt J, Apfelbacher C, Spuls PI, et al. The harmonizing outcome measures for eczema (HOME) roadmap: a methodological framework to develop core sets of outcome measurements in dermatology. J Invest Dermatol 2015;135:24–30.
5. Hoare C, Li Wan Po A, Williams H. Systematic review of treatments for atopic eczema. Health Technol Assess 2000;4:1–191.
6. Eichenfield LF, Tom WL, Berger TG, et al. Guidelines of care for the management of atopic dermatitis: section 2. Management and treatment of atopic dermatitis with topical therapies. J Am Acad Dermatol 2014;71:116–32.
7. Sidbury R, Davis DM, Cohen DE, et al. Guidelines of care for the management of atopic dermatitis: section 3. Management and treatment with phototherapy and systemic agents. J Am Acad Dermatol 2014;71:327–49.
8. Huang JT, Abrams M, Tlougan B, et al. Treatment of staphylococcus aureus colonization in atopic dermatitis decreases disease severity. Pediatrics 2009;123:e808–14.
9. Akerstrom U, Reitamo S, Langeland T, et al. Comparison of moisturizing creams for the prevention of atopic dermatitis relapse: a randomized double-blind controlled multicentre clinical trial. Acta Derm Venereol 2015;95:587–92.
10. Berth-Jones J, Damstra RJ, Golsch S, et al. Twice weekly fluticasone propionate added to emollient maintenance treatment to reduce risk of relapse in atopic dermatitis: randomised, double blind, parallel group study. BMJ 2003;326:1367.
11. Fukuie T, Hirakawa S, Narita M, et al. Potential preventive effects of proactive therapy on sensitization in moderate to severe childhood atopic dermatitis: a randomized, investigator-blinded, controlled study. J Dermatol 2016;43(11):1283–92.
12. Glazenburg EJ, Wolkerstorfer A, Gerretsen AL, et al. Efficacy and safety of fluticasone propionate 0.005% ointment in the long-term maintenance treatment of children with atopic dermatitis: differences between boys and girls? Pediatr Allergy Immunol 2009;20:59–66.
13. Hanifin J, Gupta AK, Rajagopalan R. Intermittent dosing of fluticasone propionate cream for reducing the risk of relapse in atopic dermatitis patients. Br J Dermatol 2002;147:528–37.
14. Kirkup ME, Birchall NM, Weinberg EG, et al. Acute and maintenance treatment of atopic dermatitis in children - two comparative studies with fluticasone propionate (0.05%) cream. J Dermatolog Treat 2003;14:141–8.
15. Luger TA, Lahfa M, Fölster-Holst R, et al. Long-term safety and tolerability of pimecrolimus cream 1% and topical corticosteroids in adults with moderate to severe atopic dermatitis. J Dermatolog Treat 2004;15:169–78.
16. Mandelin J, Remitz A, Virtanen H, et al. One-year treatment with 0.1% tacrolimus ointment versus a

corticosteroid regimen in adults with moderate to severe atopic dermatitis: a randomized, double-blind, comparative trial. Acta Derm Venereol 2010;90:170–4.

17. Peserico A, Stadtler G, Sebastian M, et al. Reduction of relapses of atopic dermatitis with methylprednisolone aceponate cream twice weekly in addition to maintenance treatment with emollient: a multicentre, randomized, double-blind, controlled study. Br J Dermatol 2008;158:801–7.

18. Reitamo S, Ortonne JP, Sand C, et al. A multicentre, randomized, double-blind, controlled study of long-term treatment with 0.1% tacrolimus ointment in adults with moderate to severe atopic dermatitis. Br J Dermatol 2005;152:1282–9.

19. Sigurgeirsson B, Boznanski A, Todd G, et al. Safety and efficacy of pimecrolimus in atopic dermatitis: a 5-year randomized trial. Pediatrics 2015;135:597–606.

20. Gollnick H, Kaufmann R, Stough D, et al. Pimecrolimus cream 1% in the long-term management of adult atopic dermatitis: prevention of flare progression. A randomized controlled trial. Br J Dermatol 2008;158:1083–93.

21. Hanifin JM, Ling MR, Langley R, et al. Tacrolimus ointment for the treatment of atopic dermatitis in adult patients: part I, efficacy. J Am Acad Dermatol 2001;44:S28–38.

22. Soter NA, Fleischer AB Jr, Webster GF, et al. Tacrolimus ointment for the treatment of atopic dermatitis in adult patients: part II, safety. J Am Acad Dermatol 2001;44:S39–46.

23. Meurer M, Fartasch M, Albrecht G, et al. Long-term efficacy and safety of pimecrolimus cream 1% in adults with moderate atopic dermatitis. Dermatology 2004;208:365–72.

24. Thaçi D, Reitamo S, Gonzalez Ensenat MA, et al. Proactive disease management with 0·03% tacrolimus ointment for children with atopic dermatitis: results of a randomized, multicentre, comparative study. Br J Dermatol 2008;159:1348–56.

25. Wollenberg A, Reitamo S, Atzori F, et al. Proactive treatment of atopic dermatitis in adults with 0.1% tacrolimus ointment. Allergy 2008;63:742–50.

26. Wirén K, Nohlgård C, Nyberg F, et al. Treatment with a barrier-strengthening moisturizing cream delays relapse of atopic dermatitis: a prospective and randomized controlled clinical trial. J Eur Acad Dermatol Venereol 2009;23:1267–72.

27. Patrizi A, Raone B, Ravaioli GM. Management of atopic dermatitis: safety and efficacy of phototherapy. Clin Cosmet Investig Dermatol 2015;8:511–20.

28. Granlund H, Erkko P, Remitz A, et al. Comparison of cyclosporin and UVAB phototherapy for intermittent one-year treatment of atopic dermatitis. Acta Derm Venereol 2001;81:22–7.

29. Reynolds NJ, Franklin V, Gray JC, et al. Narrowband ultraviolet B and broad-band ultraviolet A phototherapy in adult atopic eczema: a randomised controlled trial. Lancet 2001;357:2012–6.

30. Bemanian MH, Movahedi M, Farhoudi A, et al. High doses intravenous immunoglobulin versus oral cyclosporine in the treatment of severe atopic dermatitis. Iran J Allergy Asthma Immunol 2005;4:139–43.

31. El-Khalawany MA, Hassan H, Shaaban D, et al. Methotrexate versus cyclosporine in the treatment of severe atopic dermatitis in children: a multicenter experience from Egypt. Eur J Pediatr 2013;172:351–6.

32. Haeck IM, Knol MJ, Ten Berge O, et al. Enteric-coated mycophenolate sodium versus cyclosporin A as long-term treatment in adult patients with severe atopic dermatitis: a randomized controlled trial. J Am Acad Dermatol 2011;64:1074–84.

33. Harper JI, Ahmed I, Barclay G, et al. Cyclosporin for severe childhood atopic dermatitis: short course versus continuous therapy. Br J Dermatol 2000;142:52–8.

34. Koppelhus U, Poulsen J, Grunnet N, et al. Cyclosporine and extracorporeal photopheresis are equipotent in treating severe atopic dermatitis: a randomized cross-over study comparing two efficient treatment modalities. Front Med (Lausanne) 2014;1:33.

35. Zonneveld IM, De Rie MA, Beljaards RC, et al. The long-term safety and efficacy of cyclosporin in severe refractory atopic dermatitis: a comparison of two dosage regimens. Br J Dermatol 1996;48(135 Suppl):15–20.

36. Schram ME, Roekevisch E, Leeflang MM, et al. A randomized trial of methotrexate versus azathioprine for severe atopic eczema. J Allergy Clin Immunol 2011;128:353–9.

37. Berth-Jones J, Takwale A, Tan E, et al. Azathioprine in severe adult atopic dermatitis: a double-blind, placebo-controlled, crossover trial. Br J Dermatol 2002;147:324–30.

38. Meggitt SJ, Gray JC, Reynolds NJ. Azathioprine dosed by thiopurine methyltransferase activity for moderate-to-severe atopic eczema: a double-blind, randomised controlled trial. Lancet 2006;367:839–46.

39. Zachariae H, Kragballe K, Hansen HE, et al. Renal biopsy findings in long-term cyclosporin treatment of psoriasis. Br J Dermatol 1997;136:531–5.

40. van den Borne BE, Landewe RB, Goei The HS, et al. Cyclosporin A therapy in rheumatoid arthritis: only strict application of the guidelines for safe use can prevent irreversible renal function loss. Rheumatology 1999;38:254–9.

41. Paller AS, Tom WL, Lebwohl MG, et al. Efficacy and safety of crisaborole ointment, a novel, nonsteroidal phosphodiesterase 4 (PDE4) inhibitor for the topical treatment of atopic dermatitis (AD) in children and adults. J Am Acad Dermatol 2016;75:494–503.e4.

42. Simpson EL, Bieber T, Guttman-Yassky E, et al. Two phase 3 trials of dupilumab versus placebo in atopic dermatitis. N Engl J Med 2016;375(24):2335–48.

43. Jorizzo J, Levy M, Luck A, et al. Multicenter trial for long-term safety and efficacy comparison of 0.05% desonide and 1% hydrocortisone ointments in the treatment of atopic dermatitis in pediatric patients. J Am Acad Dermatol 1995;33:74–7.

44. Thomas KS, Armstrong S, Avery A, et al. Randomised controlled trial of short bursts of a potent topical corticosteroid versus prolonged use of a mild preparation for children with mild or moderate atopic eczema. BMJ 2002;324:1–7.

45. Kapp A, Papp K, Bingham A, et al. Long-term management of atopic dermatitis in infants with topical pimecrolimus, a nonsteroid anti-inflammatory drug. J Allergy Clin Immunol 2002;110:277–84.

46. Meurer M, Fölster-Holst R, Wozel G, et al. Pimecrolimus cream in the long-term management of atopic dermatitis in adults: a six-month study. Dermatology 2002;205:271–7.

47. Paller AS, Eichenfield LF, Leung DY, et al. A 12-week study of tacrolimus ointment for the treatment of atopic dermatitis in pediatric patients. J Am Acad Dermatol 2001;44:S47–57.

48. Paller AS, Eichenfield LF, Kirsner RS, et al. Three times weekly tacrolimus ointment reduces relapse in stabilized atopic dermatitis: a new paradigm for use. Pediatrics 2008;122:e1210–8.

49. Breneman D, Fleischer AB, Abramovits W, et al. Intermittent therapy for flare prevention and long-term disease control in stabilized atopic dermatitis: a randomized comparison of 3-times-weekly applications of tacrolimus ointment versus vehicle. J Am Acad Dermatol 2008;58:990–9.

50. Ruer-Mulard M, Aberer W, Gunstone A, et al. Twice-daily versus once-daily applications of pimecrolimus cream 1% for the prevention of disease relapse in pediatric patients with atopic dermatitis. Pediatr Dermatol 2009;26:551–8.

51. Siegfried E, Korman N, Molina C, et al. Safety and efficacy of early intervention with pimecrolimus cream 1% combined with corticosteroids for major flares in infants and children with atopic dermatitis. J Dermatolog Treat 2006;17:143–50.

52. Sigurgeirsson B, Ho V, Ferrándiz C, et al. Effectiveness and safety of a prevention-of-flare-progression strategy with pimecrolimus cream 1% in the management of paediatric atopic dermatitis. J Eur Acad Dermatol Venereol 2008;22:1290–301.

53. Thaci D, Chambers C, Sidhu M, et al. Twice-weekly treatment with tacrolimus 0.03% ointment in children with atopic dermatitis: clinical efficacy and economic impact over 12 months. J Eur Acad Dermatol Venereol 2010;24:1040–6.

54. Wahn U, Bos JD, Goodfield M, et al. Efficacy and safety of pimecrolimus cream in the long-term management of atopic dermatitis in children. Pediatrics 2002;110:e2.

Special Considerations for Therapy of Pediatric Atopic Dermatitis

Nanette B. Silverberg, MD[a],*, Carola Durán-McKinster, MD[b]

KEYWORDS

- Atopic dermatitis • Seborrheic dermatitis • Atopic march • Pityriasis alba • Eczema coxsackium
- Eczema herpeticum

KEY POINTS

- Atopic dermatitis (AD) is a chronic inflammatory skin and multisystem disease that affects children differently in different age categories.
- Consideration for the presence of comorbidities is important in caring for the pediatric AD patient.
- Infantile AD can be complicated by overlap with irritant contact dermatitis and seborrheic dermatitis.
- School-aged children with AD often suffer intercurrent infections with viral and bacterial pathogens.
- Teenagers with AD may have impaired body images and are more prone to specific types of allergic contact dermatitis.

INTRODUCTION

Atopic dermatitis (AD) is a multisystem inflammatory disorder that exists within the spectrum of diseases of atopy, that is AD, food and environmental allergies, and asthma, all of which are becoming more prevalent. Most atopic diseases begin in childhood, with 85% of AD cases starting by age 5 years and about one-quarter of children experiencing wheezing or eczema symptoms by their late teen years.[1,2] The prevalence of atopic illnesses has increased 2- to 5-fold since the 1960s in developing countries in children and adolescents, with a recent estimate of 17.2% in 5- to 9-year-old children from Oregon.[3–5] Mirroring this, asthma was noted to have a prevalence rising from the 1960s to the 1980s of 183 to 284 per 100,000, with the increase being accounted for by children ages 1 to 14 years, and especially increased for children with a parent who has had asthma.[6,7] AD has a wide reaching effect on childhood and quality of life can be negatively impacted in pediatric AD, mirroring the severity noted with other pediatric chronic illnesses, such as renal disease and cystic fibrosis.[8,9]

The increased prevalence of allergic illness has been accompanied by an increase in disease persistence, especially of severe AD, into the adult years. Factors associated with persistence are onset after 2 years of age and ongoing symptomatology for 10 or more years and females in meta-analysis[10]; therefore, it is crucial that we consider not just the youngest patients with AD, but the adolescent with long-standing disease, who may have ongoing symptoms for a lifetime.

Disclosure: Dr N. Silverberg has relevant disclosure of consulting and or investigative work for Anacor/Pfizer and Astellas.

[a] Department of Dermatology, Mt Sinai St Luke's-Roosevelt Hospital Center, 1090 Amsterdam Avenue, Suite 11B, New York, NY 10025, USA; [b] Department of Pediatric Dermatology, National Institute of Pediatrics, Insurgentes Sur 3700-C, Insurgentes Cuicuilco, México City 04530, México
* Corresponding author.
E-mail address: nsilverb@chpnet.org

Dermatol Clin 35 (2017) 351–363
http://dx.doi.org/10.1016/j.det.2017.02.008
0733-8635/17/© 2017 Elsevier Inc. All rights reserved.

This article is divided into practical categories in AD based on the age/developmental time period of the child, that is: (1) infancy, (2) toddler years, (3) preschool and school-aged children, and (4) preteens and adolescents. The focus is kept on the clinical nuances of the disease, and comorbidities expected for age and treatment considerations both in prescribing and side effect profiles, with an ultimate goal to improve care and, therefore, quality of life in pediatric patients with AD.

INFANCY
Clinical Nuances

This brief overview includes common features noted in infancy that impact diagnosis and therapeutic considerations. The clinical nuances overlap with comorbidities, but are reviewed in only 1 section in the interest of space.

AD is defined as a pruritic eczematous condition with a chronic, relapsing course and a typical pattern of appearance, in infancy and early childhood of "facial, neck and extensor involvement," and often accompanied by early age of onset, xerosis, and other forms of atopy.[11] Eczematous plaques in infancy can occur anywhere, but are largely limited to the face and extensor extremities. Infants often scratch incessantly and before having the dexterity to scratch they will often rub or wiggle against surfaces to address itch. This action can be paired with significant sleep disturbance, especially in winter months when household heating decreases the relative humidity. Severity can range from a few limited plaques to erythrodermic appearance, which should be carefully differentiated from immunodeficiencies such as Leiner's disease.[12] Widespread disease in infancy is not uncommon owing to the impaired skin barrier and the thinner stratum corneum layer, allowing greater exposure to irritants and allergens. This phenomenon is reflected in clinical studies by an increased transepidermal water loss.[13]

Although recent guidelines indicate that AD should be diagnosed in the exclusion of irritant contact dermatitis (ICD), allergic contact dermatitis (ACD), and seborrheic dermatitis (SD; **Fig. 1**),[11] they do in fact overlap at times and these conditions may be more common in a child with AD or a predisposition to AD. AD is aggravated by skin contact with chemical and/or physical irritants such as excessive washing, soaps, and detergents.[14] Facial AD in infancy (**Fig. 2**) is generally complicated by an overlap with ICD caused by drool (aggravated with teething), messy eating, and the need for cleaning the face. Reduced indoor humidity can aggravate head

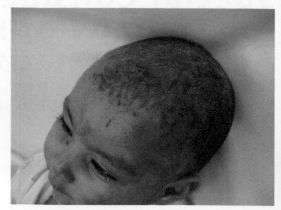

Fig. 1. Infant with atopic dermatitis and overlapping seborrheic dermatitis of the scalp.

and neck AD.[15] Facial AD in infancy is usually associated with cheek eczematous plaques. The presence of lesions on the lower cheek, where the saliva might pool, or under a pacifier, may point to a larger component of ICD.

SD may overlap with AD in infancy and it has long been felt that the overlap is not random. Alexopoulos and colleagues[16] have recently demonstrated that there is a true linkage of the 2 conditions. In their review of 87 children diagnosed

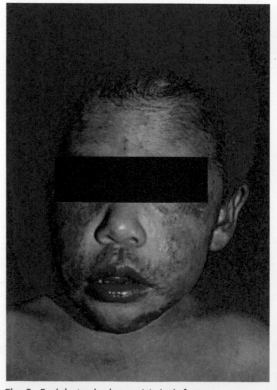

Fig. 2. Facial atopic dermatitis in infancy.

with infantile SD (ISD) (mean age, 3.1 months), they were able to follow 49 children for 5 years, with 30 developing AD features at a later age—7 diagnosed with AD concurrent to ISD and 23 diagnosed with AD on average 6.4 months after ISD onset.[16] The notable 3-fold increase in AD prevalence among ISD patients in this cohort highlights the fact that these 2 conditions cannot be separated and, as reviewed elsewhere in this article, therapy for AD, especially emollient-based care and irritant avoidance, should be initiated at ISD diagnosis. ISD in infancy often involves the skin folds as well, with maceration of the neck, and antecubital and popliteal areas, sites known to be affected by AD in older children. Yeast species including candida and *Malassezia furfur* can be isolated in these cases; therefore, the addition of an antifungal with candida coverage may benefit young children with AD and intertriginous disease.[17]

There are a series of associations of infantile AD with environmental exposures that has been explored recently in the literature. Some of the environmental associations have included pesticide exposure, laminated wood floors, carpeting, urban environment, and home mold.[18] Additionally, maternal food allergy and allergic disease, prenatal antibiotics, and prenatal stress may contribute to infantile AD occurrence.[19,20] Ultimately, it seems that some activities such as nesting or redecorating may contribute to disease triggering in the susceptible infant.

Comorbidities

The original Hanifin and Rajka criteria[21] included a list of almost 2 dozen minor features that have variable presence in childhood, depending on the age of the patient. A number of these minor criteria are comorbidities of disease. Those that are of significant concern in infancy include ISD and ICD (both discussed elsewhere in this article), food allergy, the Atopic March, and prurigo. Comorbidities of AD have recently been discussed in recent American Academy of Dermatology guidelines, which state that "Physicians should be aware of and assess for conditions associated with atopic dermatitis, such as rhinitis/rhinoconjunctivitis, asthma, food allergy, sleep disturbance, depression, and other neuropsychiatric conditions, and it is recommended that physicians discuss them with the patient as part of the treatment/management plan, when appropriate," with a level of evidence of I, II (strength of recommendation C). An integrated, multidisciplinary approach was given level of evidence III with C strength of recommendation in

the same guidelines; however, most children with severe AD do require integrated care.[22]

Food allergy
A recent US-based study looking at the effect of early introduction of topical corticosteroids with or without pimecrolimus (initially blinded and then with open-label application) as a primary prevention of the atopic march in children 3 to 18 months of age with mild to moderate AD looked at the incidence of food allergies in this population. By the end of study, 15.9% had developed at least 1 food allergen, namely, peanut (6.6%), cow's milk (4.3%), and egg white (3.9%); seafood, soybean, and wheat allergies were rare.[23] A single recent study (the LEAP trial [Induction of Tolerance Through Early Introduction of Peanut in High-Risk Children]) has identified a 4- to 5-fold reduction in peanut protein allergy since age 5 years with early peanut protein; however, allergen screen and introduction are best conducted with an allergist in the setting of known or suspected peanut allergy.[24,25] Avoidance of known food allergens in skin care products is advised as well in the setting of situations where there is an unknown refinement process and the presence or absence of the allergenic component is unknown.[26] Food allergy testing is generally performed in infants with AD when there is (1) severe disease and/or persistent disease poorly responsive to topical care or (2) known food triggers.[27] We further recommend allergy testing in the setting of potentially problematic nutrition issues owing to restrictive diets. Restrictive diets have not been recommended in the management of moderate to severe AD in the absence of proven allergens.[27]

The atopic march
The atopic march refers to the theory that AD in childhood and the associated abnormal skin barrier may allow for the development of food allergy and asthma, that is, a march from the skin to other forms of atopy.[28] The theory has some supporting evidence, although it may not describe or occur in all patients.

A variety of studies have looked at the atopic march in childhood from alternative perspectives. For example, a recent study supports the idea that percutaneous sensitization to foods may play a role in AD children, owing to an impaired skin barrier. Household dust has been identified as a potential source of peanut protein sensitization in children ages 3 to 15 months. The exposure–response relationship between peanut protein levels in household dust and peanut skin prick test sensitization is noted especially in children with a history of AD (odds ratio, 1.97;

95% confidence interval, 1.26–3.09; $P<.01$) and severe AD (odds ratio, 2.41; 95% confidence interval, 1.30–4.47; $P<.01$).[29]

The Stop Atopic March trial, a 6-year study that addressed the concept of tight AD skin control in infants as a means of allergy prevention, compared 3- to 18-month-old infants who for 3 years enrolled in a double-blind study in which they were randomized to pimecrolimus or vehicle and later received 3 years of open-label pimecrolimus. The observed mean was 2.8 years and there were no differences between the groups, with 37% developing comorbidities: asthma (10.7%), allergic rhinitis (22.4%), food allergy (15.9%), and allergic conjunctivitis (14.1%). Because both study arms offered fair disease control and barrier repair, it may be that the study design was not adequate to reveal potential therapeutic interventions needed to truly stop the atopic march.[30]

Topical and Oral Medication Risks and Benefits

Topical emollients and gentle skin care

The abnormal skin barrier in infants with AD is of particular concern owing to the intrinsically thinner skin and great irritation risk within the infantile age group, noted largely owing to incomplete barrier development at birth.[31] One of the most elucidating studies of the past few years has been a clinical trial offering at risk infants (1 parent with AD) emollient versus no emollient daily from early infancy (by 3 weeks of age) and onward. At 6 months, the intervention resulted in approximately 50% reduction in AD.[32] Furthermore, many groups have highlighted the need to avoid fragrance in at risk or AD infants.[11,32,33] Recent guidelines from the American Academy of Pediatrics subsection on dermatology have recommended every 2 to 3 days bathing for 10 to 15 minutes, lukewarm water, gentle cleanser (fragrance-free Syndet or moisturizer enhanced), and daily emollient use.[33] This is the cornerstone of therapy throughout life. Additionally fragrance-free, dye-free detergents, humidification for indoor heated homes, and cooling the home in hot summer months may enhance care.[11,33]

The eczema action plan

The eczema action plan is a goal-directed direction sheet that helps parents to recount the discussion of the office visit regarding skin care and preventive measures as well as to empower parents to initiate treatments at the first sign of flare. There are approximately 10 parameters that may be included in these documents: (1) cleansing techniques and choice of cleansers, (2) application of standard topical agents, one for the face/groin and one for the body, (3) rescue medication (a stronger topical therapy for resistant areas), (4) emollient application, (5) oral antihistamines use, (6) use of topical antibacterial agents including mupirocin and bleach baths, (7) detergent choice and clothing/fabric type, (8) control of temperature and humidity, (9) oral antibiotics when needed, and (10) other considerations, including sunscreens, allergen avoidance, and avoiding individuals with cold sores.[34] A variety of resources exist online that demonstrate potential eczema action plans ranging from flare reduction plans to global skin care plans, all of which may be used by practitioners to enhance communication and compliance.[33,35,36]

Topical medications

The topical therapy of infantile AD is largely management of the disease using the lowest potency topical corticosteroid to reduce and eliminate the localized disease flare. This generally means the use of class 5 or 6 topical corticosteroids for the face and intertriginous areas and class 3 or 4 topical corticosteroids for nonfacial areas. Rescue medication with a class 2 corticosteroid may be used occasionally, especially for severe flares of disease.

Risks in infancy include inadequate clearance, induction of parental corticosteroid phobia, and less commonly the true side effects of topical corticosteroids, including absorption and hypothalamic–pituitary–adrenal axis suppression, growth suppression, atrophy, and cataracts. Topical calcineurin inhibitors that are labeled as not intended for use under the age of 2 years have been endorsed as having evidence in support of their use for children under the age of 2 years who do not respond to topical corticosteroids.[11] There are now some published data on the safety of pimecrolimus 1% cream in particular for children with AD for 5 years, that supports infantile use through early childhood.[37]

The black box warning on the medications indicates a theoretic risk of skin cancer and lymphomas with topical calcineurin inhibitors, which may concern some parents greatly and prevent their use accordingly.[11]

Topical mupirocin 2% ointment is not a primary therapy for AD, but can be used in children with concomitant bacterial superinfection of the skin and AD and has been paired with oral antibiotics and activities such as bleach baths to prevent recurrent bacterial superinfection in AD.[11,33,38,39]

Oral medications

Oral medications have a place in all age groups of pediatric AD. On occasion, oral cyclosporine is used; however, the vast majority of children in the infantile age group are managed with topical agents and concomitant allergy screening/intervention. Oral antihistamines are used to promote somnolence in children with severe pruritus in association with AD. Sedating antihistamines include diphenhydramine and hydroxyzine. Dosage increases owing to relative reduction in efficacy should be avoided and avoidance in asthmatics with active symptoms owing to the risk of respiratory suppression is recommended. Paradoxic hyperreactivity is most frequent in younger children and signals the need to avoid the class of sedating antihistamines.

Oral antibiotics should only be used in the setting of extensive skin weeping, oozing, and/or pus discharge paired with a positive culture (usually *Staphylococcus* or *Streptococcus*). In this setting, antibiotics such as cephalexin or oxacillin that have dual *Staphylococcus* or *Streptococcus* coverage are desirable, and cultures should be performed to identify potential need for therapy of methicillin-resistant *Staphylococcus aureus*.[38,39]

TODDLERS
Clinical Nuances

AD clinical manifestations varies with age. Although dermatitis involving the face, trunk, and/or extensor extremities predominates in infants, flexural surfaces like the wrists/ankles and antecubital/popliteal fossae are more common in toddlers and preschool- and school-aged children. It may also present with other features.[40] The knowledge of the prevalence of less common clinical manifestations of AD according to age in different populations might be helpful in diagnosing incipient cases of AD.

Dennie–Morgan fold
Toddlers and preschool children may present with a Dennie–Morgan fold, a gross infraorbital fold caused by repeated scratching and rubbing of the face. It is considered by Hanifin and Rajka a minor criteria and should suggest atopy at first sight.[21] Although this finding can be linked to allergic conjunctivitis, it is in fact noted more commonly in children of color, irrespective of the presence of AD and/or allergic conjunctivitis.

Diaper dermatitis
In infants, the "diaper area" (**Fig. 3**) is often triggered by frequent cycles of skin wetting and drying as well as exposure to endogenous (eg, drool, urine, and feces) or exogenous irritants (eg, cleansing products or components of the elastic border of diapers). The latter are more common in toddlers with ACD.[41]

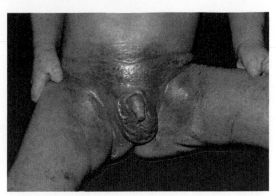

Fig. 3. Infant with known atopic dermatitis who developed diaper dermatitis.

Comorbidities
Irritant contact dermatitis
In pediatric patients, ICD is most common on the face, dorsal aspect of the hands, and "diaper area," often triggered by frequent cycles of skin wetting and drying. The most effective way to alleviate ICD is with strict avoidance of likely triggers. When triggers cannot be identified or avoided, or there is residual dermatitis after triggers have been removed, mild topical corticosteroids may reduce inflammation.

Eczema Coxsackium
Eczema Coxsackium was reported in 2013, attributable to Coxsackievirus A6, and is being recognized increasingly. In contrast with the oral erosions and gray–white, oval vesicles on the hands, feet, and buttocks typically associated with hand–foot–mouth disease, eczema Coxsackium manifests as hemorrhagic vesicles within dermatitic skin.[42] Children with AD typically have associated fever and constitutional symptoms as well as subsequent onychomadesis.[42,43] A diagnosis of eczema Coxsackium is confirmed by serum polymerase chain reaction for Coxsackievirus. Treatment is supportive, with antipyretics and bland skin care.

Perianal bacterial dermatitis
Perianal streptococcal dermatitis, predominantly affecting children and particularly younger children, is most commonly caused by group A beta-hemolytic streptococci. The clinical picture of a sharply demarcated perianal erythema is very characteristic. The diagnosis is made by either a swab of the affected region submitted for microbiological analysis with the specific question for group A beta-hemolytic streptococci, or a rapid strep test. Systemic antibiotics such as penicillin, erythromycin, newer macrolides, or others, probably augmented by topical antiseptic or

antibiotic ointments, are the treatment of choice. Treatment duration should be at least 14 days or, even better, 21 days, and be dictated by clinical and microbiological cure.[44] Recently in the United States there has been a notable increase in perineal and perianal *S aureus* infection with dermatitis, often associated with AD. These cases sometimes have mixed *Staphylococcus* and *Streptococcus* overgrowth and present with less sharply demarcated lesions and more pruritus and eczematous changes. Culture becomes important; however, milder cases of the latter can be treated like superinfected AD.[45]

Topical and Oral Medication Risks and Benefits

Nuances in topical therapeutics for toddlers and school-aged children are similar to toddlers, with the exception of the cases as noted. Specific review of therapeutics for unusual presentations was reviewed elsewhere in this article.

PRESCHOOL AND SCHOOL-AGED CHILDREN
Clinical Nuances

Pityriasis alba
Pityriasis alba is a common, idiopathic asymptomatic condition. Pityriasis alba is associated with AD as a minor diagnostic criterion. Pityriasis alba is most often present in school-aged children with no gender bias.[46] Poorly circumscribed, hypopigmented patches are most often on the face and proximal upper extremities. Patches become more prominent during summer sun exposure as the surrounding skin tans, and it is more apparent on darker skin tones.[46] In winter, hypopigmentation is less prominent. Emollients can minimize scaling, but will not impact hypopigmentation, which may persist for months despite control of xerosis. A few reports have documented efficacy of pimecrolimus cream 1%[47]

Nummular dermatitis
Nummular dermatitis is characterized by well-demarcated round or oval plaques (ie, nummular), usually asymmetrically distributed on the limbs (**Fig. 4**). Unlike typical AD, nummular dermatitis is unusual before age 5 and itch is not a common symptom.[48] The cause of nummular dermatitis is unknown, but because many cases are associated with microtrauma (eg, insect bite, scratching), and other suspected factors which include *S aureus* colonization, contact allergens, or irritants and xerosis.

Foot dermatitis
Juvenile plantar dermatosis (JPD), found mainly in children between the ages of 3 and 14 years of

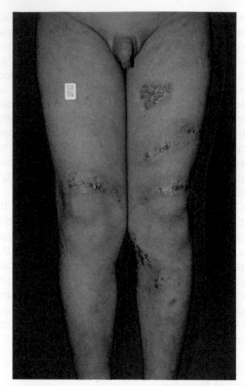

Fig. 4. Nummular dermatitis.

age, is a frictional contact dermatitis of the forefoot to which atopics are prone. The etiology of JPD is probably multifactorial. Atopy, frictional factors, and the frequent alternation between a hot and wet microclimate and a dry one seem to favor the dermatosis. JPD is characterized by dry, redness, and scaling of the feet. An ACD can also cause secondary deterioration of existing JPD.[49]

Prurigo
Prurigo has been reported in association with AD in childhood.[50] Prurigo is a manifestation of persistent uncontrolled pruritus and can be aggravated in AD by contact allergy and arthropod bites.[51] In a study in a more tropical environment—Lomé (Togo) from March to June 2013 conducted in 4 health facilities reviewed 476 children ages 0 to 15 years of age coming in for vaccination and/or pediatrics visit—31.3% were diagnosed with AD (mean age, 33.91 ± 37.0 months). AD was associated in multivariate analysis with prurigo (adjusted odds ratio, 15.59; 95% confidence interval, 7.54–32.21), allergic rhinitis (adjusted odds ratio, 7.51; 95% confidence interval, 4.31–13.10), and food allergy (adjusted odds ratio, 5.32; 95% confidence interval, 1.20–23.48).[52] Prurigo has been reported in infancy and onward, especially in studies of pediatric AD in warm climates, with a peak in preschool or school-aged children.[40]

Comorbidities

Impetigo

Impetigo is a superficial, cutaneous bacterial infection that most often occurs at sites of minor skin trauma as dermatitis. Impetigo is most often caused by *S aureus* or *Streptococcus pyogenes* and is characterized by erythema, edema, and tenderness, often with honey yellow crusting. Less common variants include bullous impetigo and streptococcal intertrigo. Pharyngeal or peri-anal *Streptococcus* carriage is a risk factor for streptococcal impetigo. Impetigo is most common in young children, but can occur at any age.[53] Patients with AD are colonized with *S aureus* on both dermatitic and normal-appearing skin. Both staphylococcal and streptococcal impetigo may be treated with skin cleansing and topical antibiotics. Dilute bleach baths may also be helpful. Oral antibiotics are indicated for widespread disease or crops of pustules. Topical mupirocin ointment may be managed with dilute bleach baths.

Molluscum dermatitis

In most atopic patients, molluscum contagiosum (MC) causes a relatively frequent infection characterized by small, umbilicated, pink, or "pearly" white papules. Most patients present a diffuse dermatitis surrounding some MC papules (molluscum dermatitis),[54] possibly owing scratching and autoinoculation to other skins sites. Bacterial superinfection can complicate molluscum dermatitis (**Fig. 5**)

Control of the dermatitis is mandatory, mainly with emollients, and to prevent spread. Data are conflicting as to the effect of topical corticosteroids on the recurrence rate.[55] Although MC is self-limiting, Harel and colleagues[56] suggests that active treatment should be offered. Curettage in an appropriate setting is very effective as revealed in a retrospective study of 2022 children with MC, where 70% of patients were cured after 1 treatment and 26% after 2 treatments.[56] Cantharidin can be used in the United States and there is extensive literature on proper technique, safety, and efficacy in children with MC.[57]

Eczema herpeticum

Eczema herpeticum, is an acute-onset, viral infection caused by herpes simplex virus. Kaposi's varicelliform eruption was used historically to refer to eczema herpeticum. It occurs almost exclusively in patients with a history of chronic AD. Patients present with widespread tender vesicles with a predilection for the areas of chronic AD plaques. Malaise, pain, and regional lymphadenopathy are often present (**Fig. 6**). With antiviral

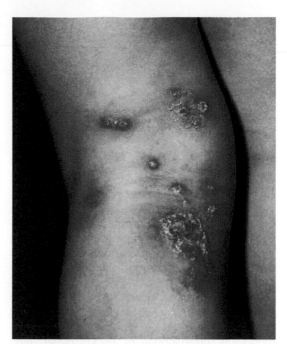

Fig. 5. Molluscum dermatitis.

treatment (eg, oral acyclovir) a quickly response is observed.[58]

Allergic and irritant contact dermatitis

Contact dermatitis is characterized by cutaneous erythema and edema. Contact dermatitis can be acute, chronic, persistent, or relapsing and it can be either irritant or allergic. In children, allergic contact dermatitis often occurs in the same distribution as irritant contact dermatitis.

ACD is classically asymmetric and geographic, following the areas of exposure to allergen. ICD is a more rapid response to physical barrier microtrauma, and is often less itchy, less geographic, and more symmetric ACD.

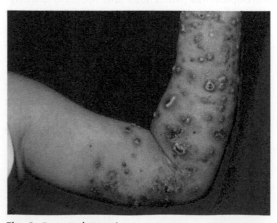

Fig. 6. Eczema herpeticum.

Both ICD and ACD commonly complicate AD. Impaired skin barrier function has been a suspected risk factor. In children with AD, contact allergy with positive patch test results were detected in 30 of 43 in children aged 1 to 5 years. Significant positive results may suggest nonspecifically positive results associated with the immaturity of the epidermal barrier during the first years of life.[59]

PRETEENS AND ADOLESCENTS
Clinical Nuances

Although traditional dogma taught that most pediatric AD clears over time, in fact, active pediatric AD may continue to flare or worsen in adolescence. Factors associated with adolescent flaring are yet to be fully determined; however, it is known that adolescent (>10 years) severity on the Nottingham Eczema Severity Score is associated with eczema onset in infancy, dust mite and food allergen sensitization, dietary avoidance, use of wet wrap, traditional Chinese medicine, immunomodulants (azathioprine or cyclosporine), high immunoglobulin E (IgE) level, and eosinophil count, but not with a family or personal history of atopy. In follow-up tracking patients from childhood to adolescence, 48% of children remained in the same severity grade, 39% improved, and 13% deteriorated.[60]

Features that distinguish AD in adolescence are a greater focus on aeroallergens, including disease of the head and neck disease, overlap with adolescent SD, increased risk of ICD and ACD aggravating or altering the clinical disease, lip licker's dermatitis, hand eczema, and JPD.[60]

Comorbidities

ICD occurs more commonly in a generalized fashion in AD. It has been shown that individuals with a lower irritant threshold in AD have increased transepidermal water loss and reduced skin hydration.[61] A variety of chemicals can induce ICD in AD, such as fragrance, and this may aggravate underlying AD. ACD is also common in AD in this age group and can be associated with aeroallergens, Malasezzia sensitization, and contact allergens, for example, lanolin. Food allergies still exist, or new ones develop with age in children with AD, but these patients often present earlier in life and it is therefore reviewed in younger age groups.

Malassezia

Malassezia overgrowth can occur in individuals at puberty and can induce proinflammatory cytokines and reactive T cells,[62] which may contribute to pubertal head and neck AD. One specific mechanism of contribution to AD activity may be Malassezia sensitization, which may result in a specific occurrence of AD in the head and neck region, in sites normally colonized with Malassezia. A risk factor for this to occur is infantile AD with food allergy. A recent study enrolled 187 infants with AD (94 children [50%] had mild, 57 [30%] had moderate, and 36 [19%] had severe AD) and food allergies before 1 year of age (49% with milk and wheat allergy, 13% milk alone, and 38% wheat allergy alone). At 10 years of age, specific IgE against Malassezia mix was positive ($\geq$0.35 kU/L) in 27%, specific IgE against M sympodialis in 20% of the 187 children. Correlation was noted with severe AD and food allergy together as a risk for sensitization to Malassezia at 10 years of age.[63] A study in adults with severe AD also reveals increased sensitization to house dust mites and M sympodialis.[64]

Allergic contact dermatitis

A recent series addressed patch test results of 349 children with and without AD (0–15 years old) over a 7-year period. Among the 349 children, 69.3% had 1 or more allergen identified, and 55.3% of children had AD. Of the AD children who reacted, dermatitis was significantly more widespread. Sensitizers included nickel (16.3%), cobalt (6.9%), Kathon CG (5.4%), potassium dichromate (5.1%), fragrance mix (4.3%), and neomycin (4.3%).[65] A second study addressing 134 children with AD via patch testing identified a 1+ reaction in 33.8% of children (n = 45). The most frequent allergen in the group was nickel (37.8%). Of the nickel-allergic children, the SCORAD (Scoring Atopic Dermatitis) was higher, as was pruritus, extent of disease, and sleep disturbance. The next most common allergens were Kathon CG (20%) and thimerosal (15.6%).[66] The importance of these recent studies is in demonstrating current contact allergen trends. These are extremely important in the preteen and teen years because children have the ability to purchase their own products in this age group. For instance, nickel is ubiquitous in belt buckles and buttonflies, but also in cell phone covers and electronic devices such as iPads.[67,68] Additionally, fragrance use increases in adolescence and continues to be a significant issue in adults with AD, especially those with facial disease.[69]

Finally, many hand wipes and make up wipes contain Kathon CG. Therefore, it may become important not only to question the parent, but also the child and further to patch test in extensive disease with an eye toward identification of an agent that when withdrawn will allow for significant disease improvement.

Attention deficit hyperactivity disorder

Data from the Taiwan Children Health Study on 2896 children with AD in the past year demonstrated a statistical association of AD with attention deficit hyperactivity disorder, Oppositional defiant disorder, inattentiveness, and hyperactive–impulsive symptoms of attention deficit hyperactivity disorder.[70] It is unclear if this is triggered by chronic itch, chronic sleep disturbance, or via an alternative mechanism; however, anecdotally one of the authors has noted some children have ewer AD symptoms when treated for the attention deficit hyperactivity disorder, this potentially being as a result of reduced impulsive scratching.

Headaches

Headaches have recently been noted more frequently in children with eczema. A combined series of more than 400,000 children and adolescents with AD showed greater prevalence and odds of headache, the highest odds being in severe AD, AD with other atopy and sleep disturbances, including fatigue, excessive daytime sleepiness, insomnia, and 0 to 3 nights of sufficient sleep.[71]

Impaired body image and coping skills

Children with AD may have a blunted opportunity to develop coping skills. Furthermore, for both sexes (but especially for girls), there are negative effects on role identity and gender role with AD. Finally, cutaneous body image may be impaired in children and adolescents with AD. Scores such as the Cutaneous Body Image Scale can be used to evaluate teens with AD. Empowerment through education and psychological intervention can benefit some children and teenagers with these specific issues.[72]

Depression and anxiety

A study of Taiwanese patients with AD assessed through the Taiwan National Health Insurance Research Database in 1998 to 2008 and demonstrated an increased risk of major depression, depressive disorders, and anxiety disorders starting in adolescence.[73]

Cataracts

Historically, cataracts were noted commonly in adolescents and adults with AD in the era before the availability of calcineurin inhibitors. A study in 1985 of 152 Japanese adolescents and adults with AD, 12.4% had an atopic cataract (n = 19), with an association with severe AD but no relationship to respiratory atopy or serum IgE.[74] It may be that the recent trend toward periocular calcineurin inhibitors for periocular AD can reduce the prevalence of the atopic cataract.

Poor socialization and coping

Restrictive socialization style in households can aggravate AD.[75] Likewise, adolescent AD patients are less likely to cope with stress in social situations and may later be at risk to develop depression.[76,77] Quality of life and coping strategies are related to disease activity in adolescence and may identify a child or family requiring referral for psychological support services.[78]

Lifestyle: sports and garments

Shoes and clothes are more of an issue for girls with AD.[79] In contrast, sports is a significant issue in adolescent males with AD. For instance, herpes gladiatorum can convert to eczema herpeticum in adolescents with AD.[58] Other issues include the risk of molluscum infection with swimming pool use, which may cause more widespread disease in AD.[80,81] As well, AD children who swim may be exposed to chemicals that promote asthma development.[82] Finally, children with AD are at greater risk for sedentary behavior, theoretically because of sweat-induced flares, and this issue may need to be addressed in the AD adolescent population as general health risk.[83,84]

Dust allergy

Dust allergy becomes more common with age in individuals with AD. A recent study looking at AD patients over the age of 3 years identified that adolescents (13–17 years) and those 18 years or older are statistically more likely to have dust allergy than 3- to 12-year-old patients with AD. The clinical pattern of AD disease in these patients is often quite typical with an air-exposed AD pattern (face, V of the neck).[85] The presence of a dust allergy in adolescence can be a predictor of disease severity.[60] Dust avoidance techniques—including dust covers for the mattress, reduced dust-accumulating household items especially in the bedroom, and air purifiers—may help to reduce dust exposure in sensitized individuals, but are not recommended as a routine measure by recent Cochrane database review, with the caveat that they did find an unmet need for intervention trials.[86]

Topical and Oral Medication Risks and Benefits

Topical emollients and gentle skin care

Emollients and gentle skin care should not be eliminated in the preteen and adolescent; however, there are specific issues arising in this age group that should be addressed. Preteens and teens are in charge of their skin care and the patient and parent should be queried separately regarding this issue. Many children in these age groups either do not bathe much, resulting in increased infection risk, or bathe with excessive duration, the latter of which is known to aggravate AD severity.[87] These extremes paired with aversion to emollient application in some individuals means tailoring care and review of bathing habits and hygiene become more important than in other age groups. Emollients such as petrolatum may become less appreciated by teenagers, and in fact may be comedogenic, resulting in unintended acne. Consequently, noncomedogenic emollient creams become the best option for facial, arm, chest, and back AD, sites of potential acne risk.[88]

Fragrance exposures increase in adolescence through adulthood, including personal care items, perfume use, body spray use, and scented items such as candles. The ongoing review of the need for minimization of fragrance exposure is necessary in adolescents.

Topical medications

The use of topical corticosteroids in adolescents is tricky. Lesions may be quite lichenified, requiring class II products and occasionally class I products. In contrast, striae are noted in a majority of teenage females[89] and sites such as the thighs and calves now become at risk for corticosteroid atrophy symptoms. Topical calcineurin inhibitors become ideal for head and neck lesions, areas resistant to topical steroids and especially in areas of steroid atrophy.[11,39]

Oral medications

Sedating antihistamines may interfere with daytime wakefulness and should be used with caution in the evening for adolescents, especially those beginning to drive.[90] Melatonin has been recently described as an alternative to sedating antihistamines in children and adolescents with AD.[91] Systemic agents are most important for the therapy of severe AD in adolescents owing to the lower likelihood of spontaneous remission and the need to intervene for quality of life and body image. Systemic agents include cyclosporine, which can only be used for a limited time period owing to risk of renal damage; methotrexate, which can be used successfully in some children with AD but requires hematologic and hepatic monitoring; and azathioprine, which has some risk of lymphomas.[92,93] Ultimately, the choice depends on the physician, the child's general health, and the risk tolerance of the family.

In cases where risk tolerance or side effect profile limit access to systemic medications, Narrowband ultraviolet B therapy can be used as a systemic treatment with good results in many patients, with the limitation of number of office visits.[94,95]

SUMMARY

AD is a complex multisystem disorder with its greatest manifestation in the skin. Therapy varies by age and developmental stage of childhood, and nuances in care should be addressed to allow for maximal disease control throughout childhood and adolescent years.

REFERENCES

1. Kay J, Gawkrodger DJ, Mortimer MJ, et al. The prevalence of childhood atopic eczema in a general population. J Am Acad Dermatol 1994;30:35–9.
2. Anderson HR, Bland JM, Patel S, et al. The natural history of asthma in childhood. J Epidemiol Community Health 1986;40:121–9.
3. Burney PG, Chinn S, Rona RJ. Has the prevalence of asthma increased in children? Evidence from the national study of health and growth 1973-86. BMJ 1990;300:1306–10.
4. Laughter D, Istvan JA, Tofte SJ, et al. The prevalence of atopic dermatitis in Oregon schoolchildren. J Am Acad Dermatol 2000;43:649–55.
5. Sugiura H, Umemoto N, Deguchi H, et al. Prevalence of childhood and adolescent atopic dermatitis in a Japanese population: comparison with the disease frequency examined 20 years ago. Acta Derm Venereol 1998;78:293–4.
6. Yunginger JW, Reed CE, O'Connell EJ, et al. A community-based study of the epidemiology of asthma. Incidence rates, 1964-1983. Am Rev Respir Dis 1992;146:888–94.
7. Klinnert MD, Nelson HS, Price MR, et al. Onset and persistence of childhood asthma: predictors from infancy. Pediatrics 2001;108:E69.
8. Beattie PE, Lewis-Jones MS. A comparative study of impairment of quality of life in children with skin disease and children with other chronic childhood diseases. Br J Dermatol 2006;155:145–51.
9. Hill MK, Kheirandish Pishkenari A, Braunberger TL, et al. Recent trends in disease severity and quality of life instruments for patients with atopic dermatitis: a systematic review. J Am Acad Dermatol 2016; 75(5):906–17.
10. Kim JP, Chao LX, Simpson EL, et al. Persistence of atopic dermatitis (AD): a systematic review and meta-analysis. J Am Acad Dermatol 2016;75:681–7.
11. Eichenfield LF, Tom WL, Chamlin SL, et al. Guidelines of care for the management of atopic dermatitis: section 1. Diagnosis and assessment of atopic dermatitis. J Am Acad Dermatol 2014;70:338–51.
12. Elish D, Silverberg NB. Infantile seborrheic dermatitis. Cutis 2006;77:297–300.

13. Kelleher MM, Dunn-Galvin A, Gray C, et al. Skin barrier impairment at birth predicts food allergy at 2 years of age. J Allergy Clin Immunol 2016;137:1111–6.

14. Akdis M, Aab A, Altunbulakli C, et al. Interleukins (from IL-1 to IL-38), interferons, transforming growth factor β, and TNF-α: receptors, functions, and roles in diseases. J Allergy Clin Immunol 2016;138: 984–1010.

15. Morris-Jones R, Robertson SJ, Ross JS, et al. Dermatitis caused by physical irritants. Br J Dermatol 2002;147:270–5.

16. Alexopoulos A, Kakourou T, Orfanou I, et al. Retrospective analysis of the relationship between infantile seborrheic dermatitis and atopic dermatitis. Pediatr Dermatol 2014;31:125–30.

17. Wananukul S, Chindamporn A, Yumyourn P, et al. Malassezia furfur in infantile seborrheic dermatitis. Asian Pac J Allergy Immunol 2005;23:101–5.

18. Xu F, Yan S, Zheng Q, et al. Residential risk factors for atopic dermatitis in 3- to 6-year old children: a cross-sectional study in Shanghai, China. Int J Environ Res Public Health 2016;13 [pii:E537].

19. Kantor R, Silverberg JI. Environmental risk factors and their role in the management of atopic dermatitis. Expert Rev Clin Immunol 2017;13(1):15–26.

20. Doğruel D, Bingöl G, Altıntaş DU, et al. Prevalence of and risk factors for atopic dermatitis: a birth cohort study of infants in southeast Turkey. Allergol Immunopathol (Madr) 2016;44:214–20.

21. Hanifin JM, Rajka G. Diagnostic features of atopic dermatitis. Acta Derm Venereol Suppl (Stockh) 1980;92:44–7.

22. Sidbury R, Tom WL, Bergman JN, et al. Guidelines of care for the management of atopic dermatitis: section 4. Prevention of disease flares and use of adjunctive therapies and approaches. J Am Acad Dermatol 2014;71:1218–33.

23. Spergel JM, Boguniewicz M, Schneider L, et al. Food allergy in infants with atopic dermatitis: limitations of food-specific IgE measurements. Pediatrics 2015;136:e1530–8.

24. Sicherer SH. Early introduction of peanut to infants at high allergic risk can reduce peanut allergy at age 5 years. Evid Based Med 2015;20:204.

25. Fleischer DM, Sicherer S, Greenhawt M, et al. Consensus communication on early peanut introduction and prevention of peanut allergy in high-risk infants. Pediatr Dermatol 2016;33:103–6.

26. Silverberg NB. Food, glorious food. Cutis 2011;87: 267–8.

27. Boyce JA, Assa'ad A, Burks AW, et al. Guidelines for the diagnosis and management of food allergy in the United States: summary of the NIAID-sponsored expert panel report. Nutr Res 2011;31:61–75.

28. Spergel JM, Paller AS. Atopic dermatitis and the atopic march. J Allergy Clin Immunol 2003;112: S118–27.

29. Brough HA, Liu AH, Sicherer S, et al. Atopic dermatitis increases the effect of exposure to peanut antigen in dust on peanut sensitization and likely peanut allergy. J Allergy Clin Immunol 2015;135:164–70.

30. Schneider L, Hanifin J, Boguniewicz M, et al. Study of the atopic march: development of atopic comorbidities. Pediatr Dermatol 2016;33:388–98.

31. Stamatas GN, Nikolovski J, Mack MC, et al. Infant skin physiology and development during the first years of life: a review of recent findings based on in vivo studies. Int J Cosmet Sci 2011;33:17–24.

32. Simpson EL, Chalmers JR, Hanifin JM, et al. Emollient enhancement of the skin barrier from birth offers effective atopic dermatitis prevention. J Allergy Clin Immunol 2014;134:818–23.

33. Tollefson MM, Bruckner AL, Section On Dermatology. Atopic dermatitis: skin-directed management. Pediatrics 2014;134:e1735–44.

34. Sauder MB, McEvoy A, Sampson M, et al. The effectiveness of written action plans in atopic dermatitis. Pediatr Dermatol 2016;33:e151–3.

35. Australasian Society of Clinical Immunology and Allergy (ASCIA). Action plan for eczema. Available at: https://www.allergy.org.au/images/pcc/Eczema_Action_Plan-2015.pdf. Accessed November 1, 2016.

36. American Academy of Dermatology (AAD). How will I know what to do to control the eczema? Available at: https://www.aad.org/public/diseases/eczema/eczema-resource-center/controlling-eczema/eczema-action-plan. Accessed November 1, 2016.

37. Sigurgeirsson B, Boznanski A, Todd G, et al. Safety and efficacy of pimecrolimus in atopic dermatitis: a 5-year randomized trial. Pediatrics 2015;135: 597–606.

38. Kiken DA, Silverberg NB. Atopic dermatitis in children, part 1: epidemiology, clinical features, and complications. Cutis 2006;78:241–7.

39. Kiken DA, Silverberg NB. Atopic dermatitis in children, part 2: treatment options. Cutis 2006;78: 401–6.

40. Julián-Gónzalez RE, Orozco-Covarrubias L, Durán-McKinster C, et al. Less common clinical manifestations of atopic dermatitis: prevalence by age. Pediatr Dermatol 2012;29:580–3.

41. Onken NT, Baumstark J, Belloni B, et al. Atypical diaper dermatitis: contact allergy to mercapto compounds. Pediatr Dermatol 2011;28:739–41.

42. Mathes EF, Oza V, Frieden IJ, et al. "Eczema coxsackium" and unusual cutaneous findings in an enterovirus outbreak. Pediatrics 2013;132:e149–57.

43. Lubbe J, Pournaras CC, Saurat JH. Eczema herpeticum during treatment of atopic dermatitis with 0.1% tacrolimus ointment. Dermatology 2000;201: 249–51.

44. Herbst R. Perineal streptococcal dermatitis/disease: recognition and management. Am J Clin Dermatol 2003;4:555–60.

45. Heath C, Desai N, Silverberg NB. Recent microbiological shifts in perianal bacterial dermatitis: Staphylococcus aureus predominance. Pediatr Dermatol 2009;26:696–700.

46. Lin RL, Janniger CK. Pityriasis alba. Cutis 2005;76: 21–4.

47. Fujita WH, McCormick CL, Parneix-Spake A. An exploratory study to evaluate the efficacy of pimecrolimus cream 1% for the treatment of pityriasis alba. Int J Dermatol 2007;46:700–5.

48. Krol A, Krafchik B. The differential diagnosis of atopic dermatitis in childhood. Dermatol Ther 2006; 19:73–82.

49. Pirkl S, Tennstedt D, Eggers S, et al. Juvenile plantar dermatosis: when are epicutaneous tests indicated? Hautarzt 1990;41:22–6 [in German].

50. Amer A, Fischer H. Prurigo nodularis in a 9-year-old girl. Clin Pediatr (Phila) 2009;48:93–5.

51. Vaidya DC, Schwartz RA. Prurigo nodularis: a benign dermatosis derived from a persistent pruritus. Acta Dermatovenerol Croat 2008;16:38–44.

52. Técléssou JN, Mouhari-Toure A, Akakpo S, et al. Risk factors and allergic manifestations associated with atopic dermatitis in Lomé (Togo): a multicenter study of 476 children aged 0-15 years. Med Sante Trop 2016;26:88–91 [in French].

53. Ortega-Loayza AG, Diamantis SA, Gilligan P, et al. Characterization of Staphylococcus aureus cutaneous infections in a pediatric dermatology tertiary health care outpatient facility. J Am Acad Dermatol 2010;62:804–11.

54. Dohil MA, Lin P, Lee J, et al. The epidemiology of molluscum contagiosum in children. J Am Acad Dermatol 2006;54:47–54.

55. Berger EM, Orlow SJ, Patel RR, et al. Experience with molluscum contagiosum and associated inflammatory reactions in a pediatric dermatology practice: the bump that rashes. Arch Dermatol 2012;48: 1257–64.

56. Harel A, Kutz AM, Hadj-Rabia S, et al. To treat molluscum contagiosum or not-curettage: an effective, well-accepted treatment modality. Pediatr Dermatol 2016;33(6):640–5.

57. Silverberg NB, Sidbury R, Mancini AJ. Childhood molluscum contagiosum: experience with cantharidin therapy in 300 patients. J Am Acad Dermatol 2000;43:503–7.

58. Shenoy R, Mostow E, Cain G. Eczema herpeticum in a wrestler. Clin J Sport Med 2015;25:e18–9.

59. Silny W, Bartoszak L, Jenerowicz D, et al. Prevalence of contact allergy in children suffering from atopic dermatitis, seborrhoeic dermatitis and in healthy controls. Ann Agric Environ Med 2013;20: 55–60.

60. Hon KL, Tsang YC, Poon TC, et al. Predicting eczema severity beyond childhood. World J Pediatr 2016;12:44–8.

61. Darlenski R, Kazandjieva J, Tsankov N, et al. Acute irritant threshold correlates with barrier function, skin hydration and contact hypersensitivity in atopic dermatitis and rosacea. Exp Dermatol 2013;22:752–3.

62. Glatz M, Bosshard PP, Hoetzenecker W, et al. The role of Malassezia spp. in atopic dermatitis. J Clin Med 2015;4:1217–28.

63. Kekki OM, Scheynius A, Poikonen S, et al. Sensitization to Malassezia in children with atopic dermatitis combined with food allergy. Pediatr Allergy Immunol 2013;24:244–9.

64. Mittermann I, Wikberg G, Johansson C, et al. IgE sensitization profiles differ between adult patients with severe and moderate atopic dermatitis. PLoS One 2016;11:e0156077.

65. Schena D, Papagrigoraki A, Tessari G, et al. Allergic contact dermatitis in children with and without atopic dermatitis. Dermatitis 2012;23:275–80.

66. Akan A, Toyran M, Vezir E, et al. The patterns and clinical relevance of contact allergen sensitization in a pediatric population with atopic dermatitis. Turk J Med Sci 2015;45:1207–13.

67. Tuchman M, Silverberg JI, Jacob SE, et al. Nickel contact dermatitis in children. Clin Dermatol 2015; 33:320–6.

68. Jacob SE, Admani S. iPad–increasing nickel exposure in children. Pediatrics 2014;134:e580–2.

69. Larsen W, Nakayama H, Lindberg M, et al. Fragrance contact dermatitis: a worldwide multicenter investigation (Part I). Am J Contact Dermat 1996;7:77–83.

70. Lin YT, Chen YC, Gau SS, et al. Associations between allergic diseases and attention deficit hyperactivity. oppositional defiant disorder in children. Pediatr Res 2016;80:480–5.

71. Silverberg JI. Association between childhood eczema and headaches: an analysis of 19 US population-based studies. J Allergy Clin Immunol 2016;137:492–9.

72. Nguyen CM. Psychodermatologic effects of atopic dermatitis and acne: a review on self-esteem and identity. Pediatr Dermatol 2016;33:129–35.

73. Cheng CM, Hsu JW, Huang KL, et al. Risk of developing major depressive disorder and anxiety disorders among adolescents and adults with atopic dermatitis: a nationwide longitudinal study. J Affect Disord 2015;178:60–5.

74. Uehara M, Amemiya T, Arai M. Atopic cataracts in a Japanese population. With special reference to factors possibly relevant to cataract formation. Dermatologica 1985;170:180–4.

75. Liedtke R. Socialization and psychosomatic disease: an empirical study of the educational style of parents with psychosomatic children. Psychother Psychosom 1990;54:208–13.

76. Sato Y, Hiyoshi A, Melinder C, et al. Asthma and atopic diseases in adolescence and antidepressant

medication in middle age. J Health Psychol 2016 [pii:1359105316660181].

77. Park H, Kim K. Association of perceived stress with atopic dermatitis in adults: a Population-Based Study in Korea. Int J Environ Res Public Health 2016;13 [pii:E760].

78. Weisshaar E, Diepgen TL, Bruckner T, et al. Itch intensity evaluated in the German Atopic Dermatitis Intervention Study (GADIS): correlations with quality of life, coping behaviour and SCORAD severity in 823 children. Acta Derm Venereol 2008;88:234–9.

79. Hon KL, Leung TF, Wong KY, et al. Does age or gender influence quality of life in children with atopic dermatitis? Clin Exp Dermatol 2008;33:705–9.

80. Olsen JR, Gallacher J, Piguet V, et al. Epidemiology of molluscum contagiosum in children: a systematic review. Fam Pract 2014;31:130–6.

81. Silverberg NB. Warts and molluscum in children. Adv Dermatol 2004;20:23–73.

82. Bernard A, Carbonnelle S, de Burbure C, et al. Chlorinated pool attendance, atopy, and the risk of asthma during childhood. Environ Health Perspect 2006;114:1567–73.

83. Smith MP, Berdel D, Bauer CP, et al. Asthma and rhinitis are associated with less objectively-measured moderate and vigorous physical activity, but similar sport participation, in adolescent German boys: GINIplus and LISAplus Cohorts. PLoS One 2016;11:e0161461.

84. Strom MA, Silverberg JI. Associations of physical activity and sedentary behavior with atopic disease in United States children. J Pediatr 2016;174:247–53.e3.

85. Dou X, Kim J, Ni CY, et al. Atopy patch test with house dust mite in Chinese patients with atopic dermatitis. J Eur Acad Dermatol Venereol 2016;30: 1522–6.

86. Nankervis H, Pynn EV, Boyle RJ, et al. House dust mite reduction and avoidance measures for treating eczema. Cochrane Database Syst Rev 2015;(1): CD008426.

87. Koutroulis I, Pyle T, Kopylov D, et al. The association between bathing habits and severity of atopic dermatitis in children. Clin Pediatr (Phila) 2016;55: 176–81.

88. Goodman G. Cleansing and moisturizing in acne patients. Am J Clin Dermatol 2009;10(Suppl 1):1–6.

89. Al-Himdani S, Ud-Din S, Gilmore S, et al. Striae distensae: a comprehensive review and evidence-based evaluation of prophylaxis and treatment. Br J Dermatol 2014;170:527–47.

90. Yu SH, Attarian H, Zee P, et al. Burden of sleep and fatigue in US adults with atopic dermatitis. Dermatitis 2016;27:50–8.

91. Chang YS, Chou YT, Lee JH, et al. Atopic dermatitis, melatonin, and sleep disturbance. Pediatrics 2014; 134:e397–405.

92. Slater NA, Morrell DS. Systemic therapy of childhood atopic dermatitis. Clin Dermatol 2015;33: 289–99.

93. Sidbury R, Davis DM, Cohen DE, et al, American Academy of Dermatology. Guidelines of care for the management of atopic dermatitis: section 3. Management and treatment with phototherapy and systemic agents. J Am Acad Dermatol 2014;71: 327–49.

94. Song E, Reja D, Silverberg N, et al. Phototherapy: kids are not just little people. Clin Dermatol 2015; 33:672–80.

95. Rodenbeck DL, Silverberg JI, Silverberg NB. Phototherapy for atopic dermatitis. Clin Dermatol 2016;34: 607–13.

Management of Atopic Hand Dermatitis

Anne-Sofie Halling-Overgaard, MS[a], Claus Zachariae, MD, DmSci[a],
Jacob P. Thyssen, MD, PhD, DmSci[a,b],*

KEYWORDS

- Atopic dermatitis • Hand eczema • Irritant contact dermatitis • Allergic contact dermatitis

KEY POINTS

- Atopic dermatitis in childhood is associated with occupational hand eczema in adulthood.
- Patients with filaggrin gene mutations have an increased risk of developing hand eczema but only in the context of atopic dermatitis.
- It is important to identify and prevent exposure to culprit irritants and allergens that may cause or worsen hand eczema.
- First-line therapy in patients with atopic dermatitis and hand eczema includes emollients and topical corticosteroids.

INTRODUCTION

Atopic dermatitis (AD), a common chronic inflammatory skin disease characterized by pruritus and eczematous lesions, affects 10% to 20% of the population.[1] The condition often begins during early childhood; although some patients obtain full remission, AD persists or relapses in many patients during adolescence and adulthood.[1]

Hand eczema (HE) occurs often in children and adults with AD.[2–4] In this clinical review article, the authors provide an overview of the most important clinical aspects of HE in AD, with a special emphasis on management.

CLASSIFICATION AND CLINICAL SUBTYPES OF HAND ECZEMA

HE is divided into various subtypes based on either cause or morphology (Table 1), and several proposals exist in the literature.[5–7] It can be difficult to clinically appreciate such complex classification because there is often no apparent link between the etiologic and morphologic picture and because the morphology of lesions, and even the cause, often change over time in affected patients.[5,7,8] Interested readers may access a clinically meaningful guideline with photographs showing the different subtypes.[5]

Acute HE is characterized by erythema, edema, and vesicles, whereas chronic HE predominantly displays hyperkeratosis, scaly skin, and fissures.[2,5] The location of HE depends to a certain degree on the different etiologic subtypes. Hence, HE, primarily located to the dorsal aspects of the fingers and hands, is a common anatomic predilection site of AD in children and adults[2] but importantly also a frequent comorbidity due to irritant contact dermatitis (ICD) and/or allergic contact dermatitis (ACD) to for example, rubber chemicals.[9–11]

The most frequent HE etiologic subtypes include ICD, ACD, protein contact dermatitis (PCD), and HE as a natural part of AD, so-called atopic HE (AHE).[6–8] According to a cross-sectional multicenter study

Disclosure Statement: The authors have nothing to disclose.
a Department of Dermatology and Allergy, Herlev and Gentofte Hospital, University of Copenhagen, Kildegårdsvej 28, Hellerup DK-2900, Denmark; b National Allergy Research Centre, Herlev and Gentofte Hospital, University of Copenhagen, Kildegårdsvej 28, Hellerup DK-2900, Denmark
* Corresponding author. Department of Dermatology and Allergy, Herlev and Gentofte Hospital, University of Copenhagen, Kildegårdsvej 28, Hellerup DK-2900, Denmark.
E-mail address: Jacob.p.thyssen@regionh.dk

Dermatol Clin 35 (2017) 365–372
http://dx.doi.org/10.1016/j.det.2017.02.010
0733-8635/17/© 2017 Elsevier Inc. All rights reserved.

Table 1
Subtypes of hand eczema

Morphologic Subtypes	Etiologic Subtypes
• Chronic fissured HE • Recurrent vesicular HE • Hyperkeratotic palmar eczema • Pulpitis • Interdigital eczema • Nummular hand eczema	• Allergic contact dermatitis • Irritant contact dermatitis • Protein contact dermatitis • Atopic HE

Data from Menne T, Johansen JD, Sommerlund M, et al. Hand eczema guidelines based on the Danish guidelines for the diagnosis and treatment of hand eczema. Contact Dermatitis 2011;65(1):3–12.

including 319 European patients with HE, the most frequent subtypes were ICD (21.5%), combined ACD and ICD (15.2%), ACD (15.2%), vesicular HE (9.3%), combined AHE and ICD (7.8%), AHE (5.8%), and hyperkeratotic eczema (5.3%).[6]

ACD is diagnosed by a positive patch test reaction and a concomitant history of exposure to the contact allergens. Acute inflammation due to ACD is often characterized by the presence of vesicles and erythema, particularly if allergen exposure is significant; but chronic ACD can be noncharacteristic with hyperkeratosis and fissures. The location of ACD normally begins at the site of skin contact (**Fig. 1**) but may spread to involve major parts of the hands, and even body, if exposure persists.[8] Traditional clinical examples of ACD include glove-related ACD on the wrists and dorsal aspects of the hands, nickel-related ACD on finger tips (pulpitis), and chromium-related ACD from cement on the palms.

ICD is diagnosed by a history of significant exposure to an irritant as well as a temporal relationship between irritant exposure and onset of HE. ICD can be located on both the palmar and dorsal aspects of the hands, the distal dorsal aspects of the fingers, as well as in the interdigital space (**Figs. 2–4**). From a clinical experience, wet workers often experience their first onset of ICD on the knuckles and interdigital space and then experience a gradual spread to the hands; but, as opposed to ACD, generalization is less pronounced. Although the risk of ICD is clearly increased in adult patients with AD, particularly those who are engaged in risk occupations,[9–11] ICD may also develop in young children who play with their hands in wet sandboxes or frequently suck on their hands to seek comfort. Notably, ICD is mostly limited to the sites of skin exposure.[8]

PCD is diagnosed by a positive skin-prick test and a history of exposure to protein-containing material, such as food that results in instant urticarial eruptions, pruritus, or erythema. Following repeated exposure to the allergenic proteins, there is a gradual development of eczema.[8] PCD is particularly common among patients who handle food professionally. The presence of PCD is often overlooked, if patch testing is not supplemented by skin-prick testing with the suspected allergens. A retrospective study found a high prevalence of AD (48.6%) in patients with PCD and in patients with other food-related hand dermatoses, indicating that patients with AD are more susceptible to cutaneous food allergen exposure.[12]

Traditional AHE is located on the wrists and dorsal aspects of the hands (**Figs. 5** and **6**),[5] where patients are exposed to cold temperatures, dry air, solar irradiation, and air pollution, all factors that may negatively affect the skin barrier and cause dermatitis.[13–15] Notably, the different subtypes often co-occur, because AHE may be complicated by ICD, ACD, and even PCD.[5] In these multifactorial cases, there is often vesicular dermatitis in the palms or interdigital space as well.

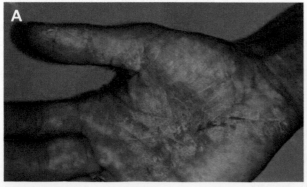
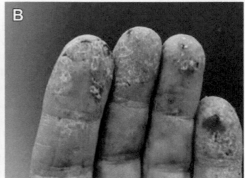

Fig. 1. (*A*) Chronic allergic contact dermatitis of the palms with hyperkeratosis and fissures caused by nickel allergy. (*B*) Acute and chronic allergic contact dermatitis on the fingers due to methylisothiazolinone exposure with erythema and vesicles as well as scales, hyperkeratosis, and fissures.

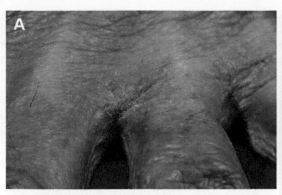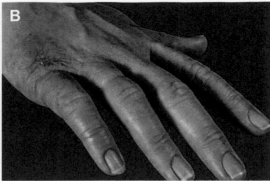

Fig. 2. (*A*) Irritant contact dermatitis in the interdigital space with erythema and scales. (*B*) Irritant contact dermatitis with spread to the knuckles following initial interdigital space eczema.

THE SKIN BARRIER IN PATIENTS WITH ATOPIC DERMATITIS

Patients with AD display skin-barrier impairment due to epidermal filaggrin deficiency caused by exogenous and/or inherited factors. These factors include a low relative humidity, excessive UV exposure, water, detergents, topical corticosteroids, and filaggrin gene (*FLG*) mutations. Epidermal filaggrin deficiency affects several important pathways, which puts further stress on the barrier.[16]

The dysfunctional skin barrier makes patients with AD significantly more susceptible to irritant exposure and increases their risk of developing ICD.[9–11] For example, application of an irritant sodium lauryl sulphate (SLS) (0.5% of SLS in an aqueous solution) result in a significantly higher skin reaction and transepidermal water loss in patients with AD irrespective of their *FLG* mutations status compared with controls.[17]

EPIDEMIOLOGY OF HAND ECZEMA IN PATIENTS WITH ATOPIC DERMATITIS

In 1985 Rystedt[18] found an association between the occurrence of AD in childhood and presence of HE in adulthood. Since then, several studies have confirmed the potent association between these clinical entities, with the highest prevalence of HE in adolescents and young adults.[2–4] Rystedt[19] showed that HE is most common in patients with AD aged 25 to 29 years, likely because of a combination of risk factors including domestic and occupational wet work.[2,20]

The association between AD and HE is strongest in patients with severe AD, in patients with AHE since childhood, and in patients with persistent AD on other parts of the body.[3,4,18] Furthermore, AD is associated with more severe HE[21,22]; the resolution of HE is less likely in patients with AD compared with patients without AD.[19] In general, studies that examined the association between AD and HE have not addressed the difference between AHE and HE due to ICD and/or ACD.[3,4,18] Although it has been a topic of

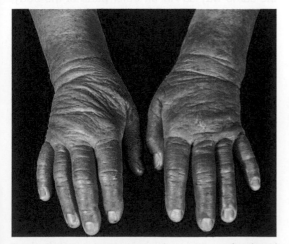

Fig. 3. Severe, irritant contact dermatitis on the dorsal side, caused by water exposure.

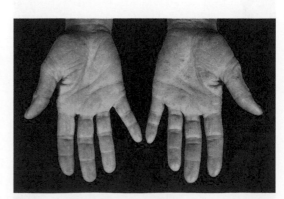

Fig. 4. Irritant contact dermatitis on the palms with typical vesicles.

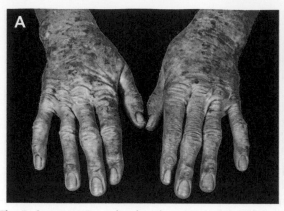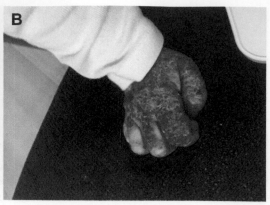

Fig. 5. Severe AHE on the dorsal aspects in (A) a patient with ichthyosis vulgaris and (B) a child with AD.

intensive discussions, it remains unclear whether AD also increases the risk of ACD; but it is likely nickel allergy and AD are associated.[23,24] It is well known that *FLG* mutations represent a major predisposing factor for AD[25]; mutation carriers have characteristic palmar hyperlinearity, xerotic skin, as well as incidental skin fissures. Epidemiologic studies have examined whether *FLG* mutations increase the risk of HE, and it seems that mutations primarily increase the risk of HE in the context of AD.[26–29] Affected patients have characteristic early onset of HE and tend to have more persistent and severe disease.[10,26,28,29]

Most studies investigating the risk of occupational HE (OHE) in patients with AD have not addressed the difference between OHE due to ICD and ACD, respectively. However, Rystedt[19]

found that 77% of OHE cases were due to ICD, whereas only 6% were due to ACD. Studies have found that patients with AD have an increased risk of developing OHE when in health care, hairdressing, and metalwork.[4,9–11,21,22,30,31] Furthermore, patients with AD tend to have more severe OHE, which results in a higher number of sick-leave episodes, job loss, and use of topical corticosteroids.[10,22] Interestingly, a recent questionnaire study found the prevalence of AD to be significantly lower among hairdresser apprentices compared with general population controls.[32] This finding indicates that patients with AD now may tend to avoid risk occupations, likely as a result of information given by physicians.

MANAGEMENT OF HAND ECZEMA IN PATIENTS WITH ATOPIC DERMATITIS

The therapy for HE is similar in patients with and without AD. Moreover, AD on the hands is treated the same way as AD on other parts of the body. Useful guidelines on AD therapy have been published, and the authors refer interested readers to these.[33–36]

Regarding the particular management of AHE, it is obviously important to first determine if there is another cause than AD (**Box 1**). A careful patient interview should, therefore, be performed whereby irritant, allergen, and protein exposure at work and home is evaluated. Irritant exposure should be quantified, for example, by the number of hand washes per work day, frequency of hand disinfectant use, frequency of glove changes per work day, and finally accumulated time of wet work, including total glove use. Also, pH and the presence of irritant chemicals in products should be examined. Protein exposure is often related to food exposure; here it is important to ask about instant pruritus, edema, and erythema following

Fig. 6. AD on the wrist.

> **Box 1**
> **Recommended management of hand eczema in patients with atopic dermatitis**
>
> - Categorize HE subtypes: morphologically and etiologically.
> - Evaluate occupational and domestic irritant and allergen and protein exposure.
> - Quantify possible irritant exposure, for example, the number of hand washes per work day, frequency of hand disinfectant use, frequency of glove changes per work day, and presence of low or high pH as well as irritant chemicals in products.
> - Identify contact allergen exposure from ingredient labels and material safety data sheets, and consider examination of products for their exact chemical content with advanced chemical analysis.
> - Diagnose possible PCD by examining whether patients have experienced instant pruritus, edema, and erythema (urticarial) following skin contact with food.
> - Assess whether resolution of dermatitis occurs over holidays and weekends.
> - Consider patch testing and skin-prick testing.
> - Educate patients in the management of HE and AD.

skin contact. Also, remember to ask about resolution of dermatitis over holidays and weekends and about episodes of sick leaves and change in job routines. Allergen exposure should be assessed by reading ingredient labels of cosmetic products (sometimes easier to have patients bring in their products), performing spot tests for allergen release (eg, for nickel, cobalt, chromium, and formaldehyde), and collection of material safety data sheets. Some clinics may also examine products for their exact chemical content with advanced chemical analysis, such as high-performance liquid chromatography.

The next step is often patch testing. Recommendations on patch testing patients with AD were recently published.[37] Notably, patch testing in patients with AD might be associated with misdiagnosing, because irritant reactions can be misinterpreted as allergic reactions.[37] If a clinically relevant contact allergy is identified, patients are recommended to avoid future allergen exposure. Similar for irritants, patients should protect their hands and avoid triggers.[8] Among patients with suspected PCD, skin-prick testing is recommended.[38]

Apart from the etiologic categorization of HE, the clinician should describe the development and morphology of HE, as it sometimes provides information related to cause. Always begin by asking where dermatitis began anatomically and how it spread to other parts. Moreover, ask for the presence of vesicles, as this could indicate ACD, whereas interdigital and dorsal location could indicate ICD; but again, there should be an exposure. It is also very important that patients are educated in the management of HE and AD. Randomized controlled trials have found educational programs to be very effective.[39,40]

MEDICAL THERAPY FOR PATIENTS WITH ATOPIC DERMATITIS WITH HAND ECZEMA

The main purposes of medical therapy are to relieve symptoms, suppress inflammation, and improve the skin barrier (**Box 2**). Therapeutic guidelines vary between countries; however, the variation seems to be small.[5,8] The combination of emollients and topical corticosteroids (TCS) represents the first-line treatment.[5,8,33,37,41] Lipid-rich hypoallergenic emollients improve the skin barrier and are always indicated in patients with AD.[5,8] Moderately potent TCS should be applied daily, often in periods of weeks to months,[5] and should then be replaced by application twice per week for a maintenance regimen.[42] However, TCS can cause atrophy, hereby limiting its chronic use. Albeit it is uncommon, patients with AD also have an increased risk of contact allergy to TCS, sometimes warranting patch testing.[43,44] It is the authors' experience that AHE, even in children, often requires mometasone furoate therapy, or a similar strength, to obtain adequate control. Topical calcineurin inhibitors (TCIs) are an alternative to TCS[5,8] because they do not cause atrophy, but they are rarely efficient in case of palmar dermatitis.[41] Coal tar represents an effective therapy that has antiproliferative, anti-inflammatory, and antipruritic effects.[45] A study found that coal tar partly works through restoration of *FLG* expression in patients with AD.[46] Coal tar can be mixed with emollients in 5% or 10% solutions and works well for nightly therapy with cotton gloves.

Eczema in patients with AD is frequently colonized by *Staphylococcus aureus*[47]; patients may, therefore, benefit from antimicrobial medicaments and antiseptic potassium permanganate baths.[48]

Box 2
Recommended medical therapy for hand eczema in patients with atopic dermatitis

- The main purposes of medical therapy are to relieve symptoms, suppress inflammation, and improve the skin barrier.
- Lipid-rich hypoallergenic emollients are always indicated in patients with AD.
- TCS is first-line therapy and should be applied daily, often in periods of weeks to months, and then replaced by maintenance therapy 2 times per week.
- TCIs can be used as an alternative to TCS but are normally less effective on palms.
- Coal tar is an alternative to TCS and TCI and can be mixed with emollients in 5% or 10% solutions and work as nightly treatment with cotton gloves.
- Patients with AD colonized with *Staphylococcus aureus* can sometimes benefit from antimicrobial therapy and antiseptic potassium permanganate baths.
- UV therapy is used as second-line therapy when topical therapy is insufficient, but it requires that patients can come for irradiation 2 to 3 times per week for 8 to 12 weeks or more.
- As last options, patients can receive systemic therapy, including acitretin, alitretinoin, azathioprine, enteric-coated mycophenolate sodium, cyclosporine, and methotrexate; but few of these are labeled for HE and AD, and efficacy is variable.

Abbreviations: TCIs, topical calcineurin inhibitors; TCS, topical corticosteroid.

A study showed that the antimicrobial therapy and a daily potassium permanganate bath significantly improved AD in patients with *Staphylococcus aureus* colonization.[48] The authors sometimes advise patients to use potassium permanganate baths for their hands 1 to 2 times per week with good results.

If topical therapy is insufficient, UV therapy (UV-B or psoralen–UV-A) can be used as second-line therapy.[5,36,41] UV therapy has many positive effects, including suppression of the immune system, improvement of the skin barrier, reduction of *Staphylococcus aureus* counts, as well as pruritus.[49] However, patients should be willing, or able, to come for irradiation 3 times per week for 12 weeks or more.

As a last option, patients can receive systemic therapy. Apart from prednisolone, which should only be used on very rare occasions, there are different medicaments available to treat AHE or other types of HE, including acitretin, alitretinoin, azathioprine (AZA), enteric-coated mycophenolate sodium (EC-MCP), cyclosporine, and methotrexate.[5,8,36,41] Alitretinoin and acitretin should in general be reserved for hyperkeratotic HE, and remember that they may worsen the already impaired skin barrier in AD. Although cyclosporine in many countries is labeled for AD, continuous treatment of extended periods greater than 1 year should be avoided. A randomized controlled trial compared cyclosporine with EC-MCP and found both medicaments to be effective in patients with severe AD; however, EC-MCP resulted in longer relapse-free periods and a more favorable

side effect profile.[50] Another randomized controlled trial found AZA and methotrexate to be equally effective in the treatment of severe AD, as about 40% in each group improved.[51] Recently, studies have examined drug survival of systemic therapy in patients with AD.[52,53] One study found that the median overall drug survival was 201 days for AZA, whereas it was 322 days for EC-MCP. Discontinuation of AZA was mainly due to side effects, whereas discontinuation of EC-MCP was mainly due to ineffectiveness.[53] Another study found that methotrexate's overall drug survival was 223 days and discontinuation of methotrexate was mainly due to side effects (25%) and ineffectiveness (15%).[52]

REFERENCES

1. Weidinger S, Novak N. Atopic dermatitis. Lancet 2016;387(10023):1109–22.
2. Simpson EL, Thompson MM, Hanifin JM. Prevalence and morphology of hand eczema in patients with atopic dermatitis. Dermatitis 2006;17(3):123–7.
3. Gronhagen C, Liden C, Wahlgren CF, et al. Hand eczema and atopic dermatitis in adolescents: a prospective cohort study from the BAMSE project. Br J Dermatol 2015;173(5):1175–82.
4. Mortz CG, Bindslev-Jensen C, Andersen KE. Hand eczema in The Odense Adolescence Cohort Study on Atopic Diseases and Dermatitis (TOACS): prevalence, incidence and risk factors from adolescence to adulthood. Br J Dermatol 2014;171(2):313–23.
5. Menne T, Johansen JD, Sommerlund M, et al. Hand eczema guidelines based on the Danish guidelines

for the diagnosis and treatment of hand eczema. Contact Dermatitis 2011;65(1):3–12.

6. Diepgen TL, Andersen KE, Brandao FM, et al. Hand eczema classification: a cross-sectional, multicentre study of the aetiology and morphology of hand eczema. Br J Dermatol 2009;160(2):353–8.

7. Agner T, Aalto-Korte K, Andersen KE, et al. Classification of hand eczema. J Eur Acad Dermatol Venereol 2015;29(12):2417–22.

8. Diepgen TL, Andersen KE, Chosidow O, et al. Guidelines for diagnosis, prevention and treatment of hand eczema. J Dtsch Dermatol Ges 2015;13(1):e1–22.

9. Visser MJ, Verberk MM, van Dijk FJ, et al. Wet work and hand eczema in apprentice nurses; part I of a prospective cohort study. Contact Dermatitis 2014; 70(1):44–55.

10. Landeck L, Visser M, Skudlik C, et al. Clinical course of occupational irritant contact dermatitis of the hands in relation to filaggrin genotype status and atopy. Br J Dermatol 2012;167(6):1302–9.

11. Dickel H, Bruckner TM, Schmidt A, et al. Impact of atopic skin diathesis on occupational skin disease incidence in a working population. J Invest Dermatol 2003;121(1):37–40.

12. Vester L, Thyssen JP, Menne T, et al. Consequences of occupational food-related hand dermatoses with a focus on protein contact dermatitis. Contact Dermatitis 2012;67(6):328–33.

13. Silverberg JI, Hanifin J, Simpson EL. Climatic factors are associated with childhood eczema prevalence in the United States. J Invest Dermatol 2013;133(7): 1752–9.

14. Kathuria P, Silverberg JI. Association of pollution and climate with atopic eczema in US children. Pediatr Allergy Immunol 2016;27(5):478–85.

15. Thyssen JP, Zirwas MJ, Elias PM. Potential role of reduced environmental UV exposure as a driver of the current epidemic of atopic dermatitis. J Allergy Clin Immunol 2015;136(5):1163–9.

16. Thyssen JP, Kezic S. Causes of epidermal filaggrin reduction and their role in the pathogenesis of atopic dermatitis. J Allergy Clin Immunol 2014;134(4):792–9.

17. Bandier J, Carlsen BC, Rasmussen MA, et al. Skin reaction and regeneration after single sodium lauryl sulfate exposure stratified by filaggrin genotype and atopic dermatitis phenotype. Br J Dermatol 2015; 172(6):1519–29.

18. Rystedt I. Hand eczema in patients with history of atopic manifestations in childhood. Acta Derm Venereol 1985;65(4):305–12.

19. Rystedt I. Atopic background in patients with occupational hand eczema. Contact Dermatitis 1985; 12(5):247–54.

20. Meding B, Lindahl G, Alderling M, et al. Is skin exposure to water mainly occupational or nonoccupational? A population-based study. Br J Dermatol 2013;168(6):1281–6.

21. Lysdal SH, Sosted H, Andersen KE, et al. Hand eczema in hairdressers: a Danish register-based study of the prevalence of hand eczema and its career consequences. Contact Dermatitis 2011; 65(3):151–8.

22. Ibler KS, Jemec GB, Flyvholm MA, et al. Hand eczema: prevalence and risk factors of hand eczema in a population of 2274 healthcare workers. Contact Dermatitis 2012;67(4):200–7.

23. Thyssen JP, McFadden JP, Kimber I. The multiple factors affecting the association between atopic dermatitis and contact sensitization. Allergy 2014; 69(1):28–36.

24. Thyssen JP, Carlsen BC, Menne T. Nickel sensitization, hand eczema, and loss-of-function mutations in the filaggrin gene. Dermatitis 2008;19(6):303–7.

25. Irvine AD, McLean WH, Leung DY. Filaggrin mutations associated with skin and allergic diseases. N Engl J Med 2011;365(14):1315–27.

26. Heede NG, Thyssen JP, Thuesen BH, et al. Anatomical patterns of dermatitis in adult filaggrin mutation carriers. J Am Acad Dermatol 2015;72(3):440–8.

27. de Jongh CM, Khrenova L, Verberk MM, et al. Loss-of-function polymorphisms in the filaggrin gene are associated with an increased susceptibility to chronic irritant contact dermatitis: a case-control study. Br J Dermatol 2008;159(3):621–7.

28. Thyssen JP, Carlsen BC, Menne T, et al. Filaggrin null mutations increase the risk and persistence of hand eczema in subjects with atopic dermatitis: results from a general population study. Br J Dermatol 2010;163(1):115–20.

29. Carson CG, Rasmussen MA, Thyssen JP, et al. Clinical presentation of atopic dermatitis by filaggrin gene mutation status during the first 7 years of life in a prospective cohort study. PloS one 2012;7(11):e48678.

30. Fischer T, Rystedt I. Hand eczema among hard-metal workers. Am J Ind Med 1985;8(4–5):381–94.

31. Lammintausta K, Kalimo K. Atopy and hand dermatitis in hospital wet work. Contact Dermatitis 1981; 7(6):301–8.

32. Bregnhoj A, Sosted H, Menne T, et al. Healthy worker effect in hairdressing apprentices. Contact Dermatitis 2011;64(2):80–4.

33. Eichenfield LF, Tom WL, Berger TG, et al. Guidelines of care for the management of atopic dermatitis: section 2. Management and treatment of atopic dermatitis with topical therapies. J Am Acad Dermatol 2014;71(1):116–32.

34. Eichenfield LF, Tom WL, Chamlin SL, et al. Guidelines of care for the management of atopic dermatitis: section 1. Diagnosis and assessment of atopic dermatitis. J Am Acad Dermatol 2014;70(2): 338–51.

35. Sidbury R, Tom WL, Bergman JN, et al. Guidelines of care for the management of atopic dermatitis: section 4. Prevention of disease flares and use of

adjunctive therapies and approaches. J Am Acad Dermatol 2014;71(6):1218–33.

36. Sidbury R, Davis DM, Cohen DE, et al. Guidelines of care for the management of atopic dermatitis: section 3. Management and treatment with phototherapy and systemic agents. J Am Acad Dermatol 2014;71(2):327–49.

37. Chen JK, Jacob SE, Nedorost ST, et al. A pragmatic approach to patch testing atopic dermatitis patients: clinical recommendations based on expert consensus opinion. Dermatitis 2016;27(4):186–92.

38. Amaro C, Goossens A. Immunological occupational contact urticaria and contact dermatitis from proteins: a review. Contact Dermatitis 2008;58(2):67–75.

39. Ibler KS, Jemec GB, Diepgen TL, et al. Skin care education and individual counselling versus treatment as usual in healthcare workers with hand eczema: randomised clinical trial. BMJ 2012;345: e7822.

40. Mollerup A, Veien NK, Johansen JD. Effectiveness of the healthy skin clinic–a randomized clinical trial of nurse-led patient counselling in hand eczema. Contact Dermatitis 2014;71(4):202–14.

41. Warshaw EM. Therapeutic options for chronic hand dermatitis. Dermatol Ther 2004;17(3):240–50.

42. Veien NK, Olholm Larsen P, Thestrup-Pedersen K, et al. Long-term, intermittent treatment of chronic hand eczema with mometasone furoate. Br J Dermatol 1999;140(5):882–6.

43. Uter W, de Padua CM, Pfahlberg A, et al. Contact allergy to topical corticosteroids–results from the IVDK and epidemiological risk assessment. J Dtsch Dermatol Ges 2009;7(1):34–41, 34–42.

44. Vind-Kezunovic D, Johansen JD, Carlsen BC. Prevalence of and factors influencing sensitization to corticosteroids in a Danish patch test population. Contact Dermatitis 2011;64(6):325–9.

45. Roelofzen JH, Aben KK, van der Valk PG, et al. Coal tar in dermatology. J Dermatolog Treat 2007;18(6): 329–34.

46. van den Bogaard EH, Bergboer JG, Vonk-Bergers M, et al. Coal tar induces AHR-dependent skin barrier repair in atopic dermatitis. J Clin Invest 2013;123(2):917–27.

47. Totte JE, van der Feltz WT, Hennekam M, et al. Prevalence and odds of Staphylococcus aureus carriage in atopic dermatitis: a systematic review and meta-analysis. Br J Dermatol 2016;175(4):687–95.

48. Breuer K, HAussler S, Kapp A, et al. Staphylococcus aureus: colonizing features and influence of an antibacterial treatment in adults with atopic dermatitis. Br J Dermatol 2002;147(1):55–61.

49. Patrizi A, Raone B, Ravaioli GM. Management of atopic dermatitis: safety and efficacy of phototherapy. Clin Cosmet Investig Dermatol 2015;8:511–20.

50. Haeck IM, Knol MJ, Ten Berge O, et al. Enteric-coated mycophenolate sodium versus cyclosporine A as long-term treatment in adult patients with severe atopic dermatitis: a randomized controlled trial. J Am Acad Dermatol 2011;64(6):1074–84.

51. Schram ME, Roekevisch E, Leeflang MM, et al. A randomized trial of methotrexate versus azathioprine for severe atopic eczema. J Allergy Clin Immunol 2011;128(2):353–9.

52. Politiek K, van der Schaft J, Coenraads PJ, et al. Drug survival for methotrexate in a daily practice cohort of adult patients with severe atopic dermatitis. Br J Dermatol 2016;174(1):201–3.

53. van der Schaft J, Politiek K, van den Reek JM, et al. Drug survival for azathioprine and enteric-coated mycophenolate sodium in a long-term daily practice cohort of adult patients with atopic dermatitis. Br J Dermatol 2016;175(1):199–202.

Adjunctive Management of Itch in Atopic Dermatitis

Sarina B. Elmariah, MD, PhD

KEYWORDS

- Itch • Atopic dermatitis • Eczema • Neuromodulator • Anti-depressant • Cannabinoid
- Acupuncture • Phototherapy

KEY POINTS

- Itch is a key component of atopic dermatitis (AD) and has a negative impact on patient quality of life.
- Reducing itch symptoms is central to disease control and may require a multifaceted approach to patient care, including barrier protection, pathogen reduction, and use of neuromodulators, in addition to standard immunosuppressive strategies.
- Currently, existing evidence to support the use of topical and systemic neural-targeted therapies is limited. Thus far, the greatest benefit has been demonstrated for opioid antagonists, topical anesthetics, and systemic antidepressants.
- Alternative therapies, such as acupuncture, stress management, and behavioral therapies, may benefit atopic patients in reducing itch.

INTRODUCTION

Itch, also referred to as pruritus, is the principal symptom of AD and its presence is essential to making the diagnosis of the disease. The severity of itch in AD ranges from mild to severe based on the degree of inflammation, the extent or site of involvement, and the chronicity of disease. Pruritus can be so intense that patients scratch until they bleed or produce scarring. Chronic itch in AD often precipitates sleep disturbance, attention difficulties, and social withdrawal, all contributing to a decreased quality of life of affected individuals.[1]

Itch sensation is mediated by activation of small-diameter unmyelinated or thinly myelinated nerves, known as C fibers or Aδ fibers, respectively, whose peripheral terminals reside in the skin (**Fig. 1**). The central projections of these afferent nerve fibers send itch signals to second-order spinal neurons in the dorsal horn of the spinal cord, which in turn project to the ventrocaudal part of the nucleus medialis dorsalis in the thalamus via the contralateral spinothalamic tract and then onto higher cortical areas[2]; see **Fig. 1**). The sensation of itch is perceived after activation of the somatosensory cortex and a subsequent scratching reflex is generated in the motor cortex and associated motor cortex. The intensity and quality of itch signals may be influenced at various points along the peripheral, spinal, and/or cortical pathways by other ascending inputs from the periphery (eg, other incoming pain or tactile or temperature-evoked sensations) or descending neural circuits (eg, influence of mood and attention).[2–4] Understanding these modulatory circuits is of particular interest and relevance in atopic itch because neurophysiologic and psychomimetric testing demonstrates that patients with AD exhibit reduced thresholds for itch and alloknesis

The author has nothing to disclose.
Department of Dermatology, Harvard Medical School, Massachusetts General Hospital, 55 Fruit Street, Boston, MA 02114, USA
E-mail address: SBELMARIAH@mgh.harvard.edu

Dermatol Clin 35 (2017) 373–394
http://dx.doi.org/10.1016/j.det.2017.02.011
0733-8635/17/© 2017 Elsevier Inc. All rights reserved.

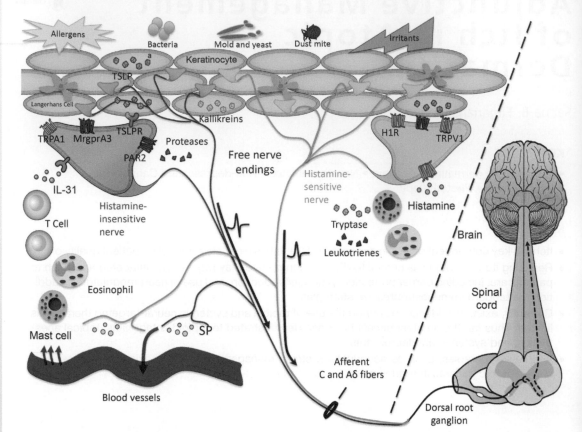

Fig. 1. Diverse pruritogens activate peripheral nerves to drive atopic itch. Sensory nerve terminals in the skin express itch sensors, known as Mas-related G protein–coupled receptors (Mrgpr); TRP channels, including TRPV1 and/or TRPA1; and protease-activated receptor (PAR) 2, all of which respond to a variety of extrinsic and intrinsic pruritogens. Exogenous stimuli (eg, irritants, house dust mite allergen, bacteria, and yeast) may directly activate the peripheral terminals of cutaneous itch-sensing nerve fibers. In atopic skin, barrier defects, such as those caused by filaggrin deficiency, result in increased release of keratinocyte-derived cytokines (eg, TSLP and proteases [eg, kallikreins]) or activation of immune mediators (eg, IL-31, tryptase, histamine, and leukotrienes) that bind directly to receptors on peripheral sensory nerves and evoke itch. Although a subset of pruriceptors also respond to histamine, histamine-evoked itch plays a minor role in atopic itch overall. Once activated, itch signals are transmitted from the periphery to the central nervous system by unmyelinated C fibers or thinly myelinated Aδ fibers, whose cell bodies reside in the dorsal root ganglia and whose central projections synapse onto neurons in the dorsal horn of the spinal cord. These spinal neurons project to second-order and then third-order spinal neurons, which ascend via the contralateral spinothalamic tract to the thalamus and onto the somatosensory cortex. Activation of peripheral pruriceptors may also elicit a peripheral feedback mechanism in which nerve endings release neuropeptides, including SP, to provoke increased vascular permability and immune cell infiltration, accounting for the erythema and inflammation observed in acute eczematous lesions.

(the ability of a nonpruritic stimulus to evoke itch) in involved and uninvolved skin.[5]

The skin-nerve interface is altered in atopic skin, with several studies demonstrating increased innervation density and expression of inflammatory neuropeptides (eg, substance P [SP], calcitonin gene–related peptide [CGRP], and vasoactive intestinal peptide in lesional atopic skin[6,7]; reviewed by Mollanazar and colleagues[8]; see **Fig. 1**). Numerous exogenous stimuli (eg, irritants and house dust mite allergens) and endogenous factors, including histamine, leukotrienes,

cytokines, proteases, neuropeptides, and many other inflammatory molecules, activate cutaneous pruriceptors (itch-sensing fibers).[9–12] The repertoire of pruritogens is expanded in AD such that nonpruritogenic and/or painful stimuli, including acetylcholine[13] and bradykinin,[14] evoke itch rather than pain.[5] Inflammatory cytokines interleukin (IL)-31 and thymic stromal lymphopoeitin (TSLP), both elevated in atopic skin, are capable of directly activating peripheral nerves to induce itch signaling in animal models.[15] Pathogenic bacteria and yeast, often colonizing atopic skin, may also directly activate peripheral nerves, exacerbating itch symptoms.[16,17]

Given the complexity of drivers that induce itch (see **Fig. 1**) and growing evidence that supraspinal processing of itch may also be altered in AD patients, the optimal approach to managing itch in AD, particularly in severe cases, must be broad and target multiple points along the itch pathway. Limiting inflammation in the skin via topical or systemic immunosuppressive therapy in patients with active eczema lesions or areas of chronic aggravation is imperative. In addition, all patients should be educated on how best to repair and reinforce the skin barrier in efforts to limit access to infection, irritants, or allergens, all of which stimulate or aggravate itch. Use of topical anesthetics or systemic neuromodulators can dampen itch signaling and may limit neural sensitization when used sufficiently early and used consistently. Moreover, limiting neuronal reflexes that trigger release of SP and other neuropeptides into the skin may reduce vascular dilatation, erythema, and subsequent recruitment of inflammatory cells. Finally, addressing physical and emotional stress is integral to an effective therapeutic regimen.

IMMUNOSUPPRESSIVE STRATEGIES

Reducing inflammatory mediators in the skin, some of which are direct pruritogens, is critical to reducing pruritus and achieving disease control in AD. The specific immunosuppressive regimen is usually determined by the severity and distribution of eczema involvement or pruritus. When localized or mild in severity, topical agents may be sufficient to control AD-related itch. Once generalized or moderate in severity, total skin or systemic therapies may be better suited to manage symptoms. Data supporting the use of these different therapies with respect to atopic itch are briefly reviewed later (summarized in **Tables 1** and **2**). A more thorough discussion of these agents and their use in AD is included in other articles in this issue.

Topical Corticosteroids

Topical corticosteroids (CSTs) have been the backbone of AD management for half a century[73–76] and remain first-line therapy for acute eczema flares.[77] Although their efficacy in treating eczema is well documented, only a handful of studies have addressed their ability to alleviate atopic itch. In a meta-analysis of 83 randomized clinical trials (RCTs) evaluating the use of topical CSTs in AD, only 39 studies investigated their effect on pruritus.[26] Of these, only 7 trials addressed itch as an independent metric; the other 32 studies included itch within the context of composite severity scores. When compared with placebo, high-potency (class 1) topical CSTs significantly improve atopic itch, often within 1 day to 4 days.[78,79] A 2012 systematic review of 6 RCTs concluded that atopic itch was reduced by approximately 34% when treated with topical CSTs of varying potencies.[80] Data regarding whether antipruritic efficacy of topical CSTs correlates with greater potency are conflicting,[81–83] although in many of these reports comparisons were made between closely related potency classes.[83–85]

Although the data overwhelmingly suggest that topical CSTs significantly improve skin lesions and pruritus in AD patients, the use of these agents is often limited due to the risk of local side effects, including atrophy and the possibility of tachyphylaxis. Due to these limitations and the frequent inability of topicals CSTs to offer complete relief to moderate to severe AD patients, alternative and systemic therapies must frequently be considered.

Topical Calcineurin Inhibitors

Topical calcineurin inhibitors (TCIs), including tacrolimus and pimecrolimus, were introduced more than 15 years ago as steroid-sparing topical agents. Calcineurin inhibitors are immunomodulators that regulate T-cell activation to inhibit the release of inflammatory cytokines.[86,87] Beyond their anti-inflammatory properties, TCIs may also mediate a direct antipruritic effect by overstimulation and subsequent desensitization of transient receptor potential (TRP) V1 ion channels on cutaneous nerve fibers.[88] In several large, double-blind, placebo-controlled RCTs in pediatric AD patients, tacrolimus ointment alleviated pruritus within the first week of treatment.[27–29] Similarly, pimecrolimus cream 1% has been shown to reduce itch within days and produces a sustained itch relief with continued use in adult and pediatric AD patients.[89–91] In several head-to-head studies, tacrolimus ointment was more effective than pimecrolimus cream in the treatment of AD, including AD-related pruritus.[92–94]

One of the most commonly reported side effects of TCIs includes a burning sensation, in part related to TRPV1 activation on cutaneous nerves.[90] TCIs do not cause skin atrophy and can be safely applied for prolonged periods on any site. Importantly, chronic TCI therapy in AD patients does not increase the risk of systemic immunosuppression, serious infections, or malignancy.[93,95–98]

Table 1
Topical antipruritic therapies

Therapy	Mechanism of Action	Supporting Evidence in Atopic Dermatitis–Related Itch	Comments
Moisturizers			
Occlusive agents (eg, petrolatum, mineral oil, dimethicone)	Prevent water evaporation	A[18–20]	First-line therapy
Humectants (eg, glycerol, lactate[s], urea, sorbital)	Attract and hold water	B[21]	—
Emollients (eg, glycol stearate, glyceryl stearate, lanolin)	Lubricate and soften the skin	A[22,23]	First-line therapy
Repair creams	*Lipid and ceramide incorporation into corneocyte scaffold*	B[24,25]	—
Topical immunomodulators			
Corticosteroids (eg, hydrocortisone, triamcinolone, betamethasone)	Activates glucocorticoid receptors that inhibit proinflammatory cytokine release	A[26]	First-line therapy; use may be limited by risks of skin-thinning, observed with prolonged use
Calcineurin inhibitors (eg, tacrolimus, pimecrolimus)	Prevents activation of the NFAT transcription factor in T cells, thereby inhibiting T-cell activation and proinflammatory cytokine release	A[27–29]	First-line maintenance
Antihistamines (eg, diphenhydramine, doxepin)	Blocks H1 and/or H2 receptors on histamine-sensitive nerve fibers	B[30]	May cause sedation with systemic absorption May cause allergic contact dermatitis
Topical antibiotics			
Antibacterial agents (eg, bacitracin, neosporin, mupirocin)	Reduces bacterial colonization, infection, and release of exotoxins	B	Cochrane review failed to show benefit in AD patients unless infected[31]
Topical neurmodulators			
Anesthetics			
Caine anesthetics (eg, lidocaine, prilocaine)	Inhibit voltage-gated sodium channels and thereby reduce the firing of nociceptive and pruriceptive sensory fibers	D[32]	Risk of allergic sensitization Prilocaine associated with methemoglobinemia in pediatric patients
Polidocanol 3%	Nonionic surfactant	B[33,34]	—

(continued on next page)

Table 1
(continued)

Therapy	Mechanism of Action	Supporting Evidence in Atopic Dermatitis–Related Itch	Comments
TRP modulators			
Capsaicin	Activates TRPV1 on sensory fibers, depleting SP over time and prevents neural transmission	B: OLS showed reduction in itch in AD-related prurigo nodularis, but otherwise controversial as antipruritic agent in AD	Burning sensation with initial use may limit patient compliance. Open label study showed reduction in itch in AD-related prurigo nodularis, but otherwise controversial as antipruritic agent in AD.
Menthol	Activates TRPM8 on sensory fibers triggering a cooling sensation	C[35]	May be useful in patients who report cooling alleviates symptoms
Cannabinoids			
N-PEA cream	Binds CB2 receptor and inhibits breakdown of anandamide; reduces mast cell degranulation	B[25,36]	—
Opioid antagonists			
Naltrexone 1% cream	MOR antagonist	B[37]	—
Miscellaneous			
Coal tar	Mechanism unknown	B[38,39]	Second-line or adjunctive therapy

A, consistent, good-quality, patient-oriented evidence, including large randomized controlled trials, meta-analyses; B, inconsistent or limited-quality patient-oriented evidence; C, consensus, usual practice, opinion, or case series; D, limited to 1 or more case reports; and E, studies showing improvement in itch but no direct evidence in AD-related itch.

Systemic Immunosuppressive Agents

Cyclosporin A

Cyclosporin A (CsA), an immunosuppressive agent used in transplant medicine since the 1970s, has proved helpful in managing several immune-mediated skin diseases, including graft-vs-host disease, psoriasis, and refractory AD.[26,99,100] Cyclosporine binds to the intracellular receptor cyclophilin, leading to decreased T-cell activation and transcription of IL-2, a mediator of pruritus.[101] Although not Food and Drug Administration (FDA) approved for the treatment of AD in the United States, it is the only immunosuppressant approved for AD in Europe. A meta-analysis of CsA efficacy in severe AD patients determined that the mean clinical improvement in disease severity after 6 weeks to 8 weeks of continuous treatment was 55%, although 50% of patients relapsed within 2 weeks.[43] Three of 15 studies included in this meta-analysis were RCTs that included itch severity as a clinical endpoint and demonstrated improvement in pruritus.[102] Additional studies have confirmed reduction in AD-related itch by 71% to 78% when CsA is dosed at 3 mg/kg to 5 mg/kg[44,45] and by 50% to 54% when dosed independent of body weight at 150 mg or 300 mg daily.[46] Careful consideration must be given to the use and duration of CsA therapy in AD in light of potential serious side effects (for example, hypertension, renal dysfunction, and hyperlipidemia.[103] Thus, CsA may best be used as a short-term solution to achieve rapid control of inflammation and itch in severe AD.

Purine synthesis inhibitors

Mycophenolate mofetil (MMF) inhibits inosine monophosphate dehydrogenase, an enzyme necessary for purine biosynthesis, and thereby

Table 2
Systemic antipruritic therapies

Therapy	Mechanism of Action	Supporting Evidence in Atopic Dermatitis–Related Itch	Comments
Antihistamines			
Sedating antihistamines (eg, doxepin, hydroxyzine)	Blocks H1 and/or H2 receptors on histamine-sensitive nerve fibers	B[40]	Improve sleep quality in AD due to sedating effects, but no improvement in itch
Nonsedating antihistamines (eg, fexofenadine, cetirizine)	Blocks H1 and/or H2 receptors on histamine-sensitive nerve fibers	C[41,42]	Despite common practice, a meta-analysis concluded nonsedating AH were ineffective
Immunosuppressive agents			
Cyclosporine	Binds to the intracellular receptor cyclophilin, leading to decreased T-cell activation and transcription of IL-2, a mediator of pruritus	A[43–46]	Limited by need for shorter duration of use
AZA	Purine analog and synthesis inhibitor, limits T-cell and B-cell proliferation	A[43,47,48]	Second-line therapy
MMF	Inosine monophosphate dehydrogenase inhibitor, T-cell and B-cell proliferation	B[49–51]	Third-line therapy
MTX	Inhibitor of dihyrdofolate reductase, which indirectly inhibits purine synthesis, limits T-cell proliferation	B[47,52]	Third-line therapy
Monoclonal antibodies			
Dupilumab	Humanized mAb that binds to and blocks IL-4 and IL-13 signaling	A[43,107]	Fast-tracked for FDA approval
Omalizumab	Humanized mAb that binds and sequesters free IgE	B[109]	Useful in urticaria and asthma
Neuromodulators			
Antiepileptics (eg, gabapentin, pregabalin)	Inhibition of voltage-gated calcium channels in peripheral and spinal nerves	E[53–58]	May be sedating
SSRIs (eg, fluvoxamine, paroxetine, sertraline)	Prevent the reuptake of serotonin into presynaptic terminals, indirectly modulating serotonergic signaling	B[59–64]	May be sedating

(continued on next page)

Table 2
(continued)

Therapy	Mechanism of Action	Supporting Evidence in Atopic Dermatitis–Related Itch	Comments
SNRIs (eg, mirtazapine)	A serotonin and norepinephrine antidepressant	B[65–67]	Less anticholinergic SE compared with SSRIs; increased risk of weight gain
Aprepitant	Neurokinin-1 receptor antagonist, blocks some actions of SP	E	Not FDA approved for itch
μ-Opioid antagonists (eg, naltrexone, nalmafene, naloxone)	μ-receptor antagonism reduces itch sensation	B[68–72]	—
κ-Opioid agonists (eg, butrophanol, nalfurafine)	k-receptor agonism reduces itch sensation	E	Nalfurafine is not available in US, used primarily in Japan

A, consistent, good-quality, patient-oriented evidence, including large randomized controlled trials, meta-analyses; B, inconsistent or limited-quality patient-oriented evidence; C, consensus, usual practice, opinion, or case series; D, limited isolated to few case reports; and E, studies showing improvement in itch but no direct evidence in AD-related itch.

prevents lymphocyte proliferation. MMF has been shown to be safe, well tolerated, and effective for the treatment of severe AD and AD-associated itch.[49,50] In 2011, Haeck and colleagues[51] reported results from an open-label trial in which 55 adult subjects with severe AD were treated with CsA for 6 weeks and subsequently randomized to either continuing CsA or transitioning to MMF for 30 weeks. Although the initial AD severity measurements were better for patients who remained on CsA, eczema severity was similar between MMF and CsA groups after 10 weeks and the duration of clinical remission after discontinuation of drug lasted longer for patients treated with MMF.[51]

Azathioprine (AZA) is a purine analog that inhibits normal purine synthesis and DNA production, limiting T-cell and B-cell proliferation. A 2014 meta-analysis of systemic immunomodulators in the treatment of moderate to severe AD recommended AZA as a second-line treatment option.[104] Several RCTs demonstrated improvement in atopic itch after treatment with AZA.[43,47,48] One double-blind RCT of 63 AD patients reported a 2.4-mm reduction on an itch visual analog scale (VAS) in subjects receiving AZA compared with 1-mm reduction in subjects receiving placebo at 12 weeks.[105] Although the potential for lymphopenia, nausea, or gastrointestinal upset must be monitored in patients taking AZA,[47,105] several studies failed to report serious adverse events after 24 weeks of treatment.[47,48,104,105]

Methotrexate (MTX), an inhibitor of dihyrdofolate reductase that indirectly inhibits purine synthesis,

is commonly used in the treatment of inflammatory skin disease[106] and has been recommended as a third-line agent for moderate to severe AD.[104] To date, there are few studies that address the impact of MTX on atopic itch. A prospective, open-label trial evaluating the efficacy of MTX in moderate to severe AD demonstrated a 52% reduction of disease severity from baseline, accompanied by significant improvements in itch severity and sleep.[52] In a head-to-head comparison of AZA and MTX, similar improvement in AD was noted in both groups, with mean decreases in itch on VAS by 2.6 mm (SD 2.2 mm) in patients receiving AZA and 2.5 mm (SD 2.2 mm) in patients receiving MTX.[47]

Monoclonal antibodies
Monoclonal antibody (mAb) therapies may also be used for the treatment of AD. Dupilumab, a fully humanized mAb that binds to and blocks IL-4 and IL-13 signaling, limits key mediators of type 2 helper T-cell allergic inflammation. In a 2013 double-blind, placebo-controlled RCT of adults with moderate to severe AD, dupilumab treatment resulted in significant and rapid improvement in all measured indicators of AD disease severity,[107] including a 55.7% reduction in itch severity compared with only 15.1% in the control group. A subsequent phase 2b dose-ranging study of dupilumab recapitulated these results.[108] Dupilumab has been fast-tracked for approval by the FDA for moderate to severe AD refractory to topical and/or other systemic medications and/or for whom such options are

contraindicated. Omalizumab, a humanized mAb that sequesters free IgE, has been approved for the treatment of patients 12 years and older with moderate to severe allergic asthma and chronic urticaria. Although a handful of case reports and small open-label studies suggest a beneficial role in AD,[109] results have been inconsistent and 1 study suggests that this variability may reflect whether or not patients carry filaggrin mutations.[110,111] The role for other therapies, including anti–IL-5 therapy (mepolizumab), anti-CD20 (rituximab), and immunoabsorption of IgE, in AD is unknown.

Phototherapy

Phototherapy is an effective, safe, and well-tolerated treatment of AD and atopic itch.[112] Although the mechanism of action of phototherapy is incompletely understood, its efficacy in treating atopic pruritus is likely multifactorial. Phototherapy reduces cutaneous inflammation by decreasing T cells in atopic skin,[113] reducing IgE-binding and mast cells in the dermis, and inhibiting the egress of Langerhans cells out of the epidermis.[114] Phototherapy also reduces the density of epidermal sensory nerves, which may contribute to a more direct antipuritic effect.[115] AD and itch are highly responsive to phototherapy regimens that span a broad range of wavelengths, including broadband and narrowband UV-B,[116,117] combined UV-A + UV-B,[118] and UV-A alone.[119] Although therapeutic benefits, including rapid reduction in itch, have been observed in AD patients after psoralen plus UV-A treatment,[120–123] potential side effects of erythema, burning, more rapid photoaging, and the risk of nonmelanoma skin cancer limit the use of this option.[124]

EMOLLIENTS/SKIN BARRIER PROTECTION

Atopic skin is characterized by a reduction in stratum corneum lipids (eg, ceramides and cholesterol)[125] and/or filaggrin deficiency,[126] both of which result in heightened transepidermal water loss (TEWL),[127] and a dysfunctional skin barrier easily penetrated by irritants, allergens, and pathogens, all of which drive atopic itch and inflammation.[128] Topical moisturizers, comprised of emollient, occlusive, and/or humectant ingredients, improve atopic itch.[18–20,22,23,129] Emollients (eg, glycol, glyceryl stearate, lanolin, and soy sterols) lubricate and soften the skin; occlusive agents (eg, petrolatum, dimethicone, and mineral oil) form a layer to prevent water evaporation; and humectants (eg, glycerol, lactic acid, and urea) attract and hold water. These ingredients work synergistically to restore the integrity of the epidermal barrier and, when used in combination with topical CSTs, improve the barrier, and reduce itch far better than topical CSTs alone.[130]

Adjunct agents routinely found in moisturizers intended to alleviate itch include colloidal oatmeal and ceramides. Oatmeal has been used for centuries to relieve itch[131] because they contain a group of phenolic alkaloids that decrease production of inflammatory mediators, including arachidonic acid, phospholipase A2, tumor necrosis factor α[132]; inhibit the activity of nuclear factor κB, a transcription factor important in innate and adaptive immune responses[133]; and prevent keratinocyte release of proinflammatory cytokines (eg, IL-8) and histamine.[133] In a recent review of studies of adjunct therapies in AD, the daily use of moisturizers and cleansers containing colloidal oatmeal significantly improved clinical outcomes, including itch severity.[134]

Ceramides, a family of waxy lipid molecules that contribute to sphingomyelin, comprise a major component of the intercellular lipids that surround keratinocytes in the stratum corneum and prevent water loss.[135,136] Decreased ceramide levels in the skin of AD patients contribute to impaired barrier function.[137,138] In a recent cohort study, a ceramide containing cleanser and moisturizer substantially improved overall disease severity and itch intensity in AD patients.[139] Consistent with this observation, moisturizers with equimolar ratio of cholesterol, ceramides, and essential and nonessential free fatty acids accelerate barrier recovery.[140] These ingredients have recently been incorporated into nonsteroidal barrier creams that integrate directly into the extracellular lipid matrix of the stratum corneum to relieve itch in adult and pediatric patients.[141–143]

Given the numerous studies that have documented the antipruritic effects of moisturizers, their liberal and frequent use should be a cornerstone of AD therapy. Patients should be directed to apply moisturizers 1 time to 3 times daily, within minutes of bathing for optimal occlusion of a hydrated stratum corneum.[144] The choice of moisturizing agent is highly dependent on individual preference, although preparations devoid of additives, fragrances, and perfumes are recommended. In addition, lower pH moisturizers are preferred in preserving barrier function and in reducing itch and irritation.[145]

ANTIBACTERIAL AGENTS

Due to a compromised barrier, atopic skin is predisposed to develop secondary bacterial, viral, and fungal skin infections. *Staphylococcus aureus* is the most common offender, reported to colonize more than 90% of adult AD patients.[146] Staphylococcus-derived exotoxins and superantigens aggravate AD symptoms and are capable of directly triggering itch,[147–149] and the density of *S aureus* colonization correlates with disease severity.[150,151] Although data regarding the utility of topical and systemic antibiotics to control colonization in AD have been controversial (addressed in a recent Cochrane review[152]) the regular practice of dilute bleach baths with concomitant intranasal topical mupirocin may be helpful for improving AD-related itch. In an RCT of 31 children with moderate to severe AD, treatment of an infectious episode with 2 weeks of oral cephalexin followed by the addition of household bleach (sodium hypochlorite) to bathwater plus intranasal mupirocin treatment for 3 months led to a statistically significant improvement in disease severity compared with placebo.[153] A prospective RCT in Malaysia showed similar results, reporting a significant reduction in itch severity after 2 months of dilute bleach baths.[154] Patients with severe itch may initially complain of irritation due to the weakly basic pH of hypochlorite in water, but this usually abates with subsequent treatments. One additional advantage of bleach over antibiotics is the lower concern for development of bacterial resistance.

ANTIHISTAMINES

Histamine is a well-established pruritogen[155] and is known to mediate the inflammatory effects of several allergic skin diseases.[156] As such, topical and oral histamines are routinely recommended by physicians to help control atopic itch. Despite this widespread practice, histamine's role in triggering itch in AD is limited and evidence supporting the use of histamine 1 (H1) or histamine 2 (H2) receptor antagonists in AD management is lacking. Emerging evidence suggests that the H4 receptor may play an important role in mediating histamine-induced inflammation and itch in AD; however, H4 antagonists are not commercially available at present.[156]

Several RCTs evaluating the effects of sedating and nonsedating oral H1 antagonists on itch relief in AD do not support substantial improvement over placebo.[157] A meta-analysis of 16 RCTs concluded that nonsedating antihistamines are ineffective in AD management, whereas sedating forms may improve sleep quality.[41] In the Early Treatment of the Atopic Child trial, infants were randomized to receive cetirizine or placebo for 18 months.[158] Although subjects receiving cetirizine had less urticaria during the treatment period, no statistically significant improvement was

observed. A dose-titrating study of 178 adults showed that a 4-fold increase in the dose of cetirizine was required to appreciably reduce pruritus, erythema, lichenification, and body surface area involvement.[159] These findings were attributed to the sedating effects of cetirizine at high doses. A small, but significant, antipruritic effect of fexofenadine, 60 mg twice daily, has been described.[42]

These data support the intermittent use of sedating antihistamines, particularly in the setting of sleep loss secondary to itch. Diphenhydramine and hydroxyzine are the most commonly used antihistamines for this purpose,[40] although some patients become tolerant to the sedating effects within 4 days to 7 days of therapy.[160] Doxepin, a tricyclic antidepressant with potent H1 receptor antagonism, is often chosen as an adjunctive agent in the management of AD because of its combined anxiolytic, antidepressant, and sedative effects. A double-blind RCT in 270 patients demonstrated significant reduction in itch after using topical doxepin 5% cream for 7 days compared with vehicle.[30] Its use, however, is limited by a high rate of allergic contact dermatitis and sedation from percutaneous absorption.[30,161] Both topical and oral antihistamines may cause sedation (including nonsedating formulations) and may elicit anticholinergic symptoms (eg, dry mouth, blurred vision, and tachycardia).[162]

NEUROMODULATORS

Consistent with the concept of AD being "the itch that rashes," a growing number of studies suggest that the nervous system is integral to promoting atopic disease in addition to mediating itch.[163] Evolving preclinical data suggest that effectively targeting the neural circuits involved in itch transmission may improve the pruritus, burning, and discomfort from which AD patients suffer. The use of neuromodulators in AD is in its relative infancy and formal evaluation of the efficacy of neuromodulation in double-blind RCTs has been rare. Despite this, preclinical and early clinical data are promising and this field will likely undergo dramatic expansion in the near future.

Topical Neuromodulators

Topical capsaicin

Capsaicin, a naturally occurring alkaloid derived from chili peppers, has been successfully used to relieve pruritus in several conditions, including prurigo nodularis, both AD-dependent and independent cases; neuropathic dermatoses; and aquagenic and uremic pruritus.[164–169] Capsaicin activates TRPV1 ion channels on nociceptors, triggering the release and depletion of neuropeptides, such as SP and/or CGRP.[170–172] Although repeated topical application of capsaicin can reduce or eliminate itch in AD-related prurigo nodularis,[168] clear evidence supporting the use of capsaicin as an antipruritic in other stages of AD is lacking.[173] One study actually demonstrated that although pretreatment with capsaicin suppressed histamine-induced itch in healthy controls, it had no effect in reducing itch in atopic individuals.[174] A potential barrier to use, capsaicin causes transient burning and local irritation. This side effect may be mitigated by preceding or concurrent application of topical anesthetics to reduce pain as well as topical CSTs to reduce initial inflammation.[128]

Topical cooling agents

Topical cooling agents have been found helpful in the management of itch and may be of use in mild AD and atopic itch. Cooling agents include menthol, camphor, and phenol, all commonly found additives in topical anti-itch lotions. Menthol and camphor are monoterpenoids that have been used since antiquity[175] and exert their effects via activation of thermosensitive TRP channels expressed by keratinocytes and peripheral nociceptors. In vitro studies demonstrate that camphor's ability to enhance the sensation of innocuous cold may be due to activation of thermosensitive TRPV3 receptors[176] and ultimately to receptor desensitization that leads to analgesic and antipruritic effects.[177] Similarly, menthol functions as an agonist of TRP melastatin-8 (TRPM8), a temperature-sensitive calcium channel expressed by peripheral afferent fibers. When activated, TRPM8 evokes the sensation of cold and can modulate the perception of pain and itch.[178–182]

Despite their widespread use in over-the-counter anti-itch preparations, evidence regarding the efficacy of these coolants in reducing atopic itch is sparse. Menthol has been demonstrated to reduce itch in patients with lichen amyloidosis and histamine-evoked and irritant-induced pruritus.[175,180,183,184] One study performed in 35 atopic pediatric patients reported that menthol spray decreased itch from baseline after 7 days.[35] Further evaluation of the efficacy of menthol and similar compounds to treat atopic itch is warranted. Caution must be advised when recommending the use of cooling agents in atopic individuals, because menthol and camphor may exacerbate TEWL.[185] Furthermore, monoterpenes may induce allergic or irritant contact dermatitis[186,187] and at higher concentrations (10%–40%) may cause erythema and burning,[188] which is of particular concern in AD patients given their compromised skin barrier.

Topical anesthetics

Topical 'caine' anesthetics have been effectively used to provide itch relief in several skin conditions.[187,189–191] Lidoocaine and prilocaine are both amide anesthetics that inhibit voltage-gated sodium channels and thereby reduce the firing of nociceptive and pruriceptive sensory fibers. In a study in 20 healthy volunteers, a mixture of lidocaine and prilocaine reduced itch evoked by histamine as well as cowhage and papain, experimental pruritogens that activate histamine-independent itch pathways.[190] Although some benefit of topical lidocaine has been demonstrated for managing neuropathic and postburn pruritus,[192–194] its efficacy in AD is limited to an isolated report in which 1 atopic patient-derived tremendous itch relief after lidocaine application.[32] Allergic sensitization to topical lidocaine must be considered, because the rate of delayed type hypersensitivity reactions is higher in prone populations.[195]

In contrast, the anesthetic surfactant polidocanol, recently shown to reduce histamine-independent itch in an experimental setting by more than 58%, has shown some promise in reducing atopic itch.[33,34] In a German multicenter, open-label trial in 1611 pediatric and adult patients with AD (47.9%), contact or other eczemas (33.7%), psoriasis (6.2%), or other pruritic dermatoses, a cream mixture of 3% polidocanol and 5% urea improved or entirely eliminated pruritus in the majority of patients.[34] Patients tolerated the topical mixture well overall, infrequently experiencing burning or itch with initial application.[34]

Topical naltrexone

Naltrexone, a μ-opioid receptor (MOR) antagonist, has been shown to reduce atopic itch in several clinical studies. In a pilot study of 18 patients with chronic pruritus of varying etiologies, including AD, more than 70% of the patients using topical 1% naltrexone cream experienced significant itch relief.[37] In a subsequent, randomized, crossover trial in AD patients, topical application of naltrexone resulted in 29.4% improvement in itch and a faster time to relief/itch reduction compared with placebo alone. Skin biopsies from patients using topical naltrexone exhibited decreased MOR expression.[37] Naltrexone and other MOR antagonists, as well as κ-opioid receptor (KOR) agonists, have been reported effective in managing intractable pruritus from multiple sources and are discussed later.

Topical cannabinoids

Palmitoylethanolamine (PEA) is an endogenous fatty acid amide with endocannabinoid-like properties that has antipruritic and analgesic effects. PEA has low affinity for cannabinoid receptors[196,197] and is thought to exert its anti-itch effects by inhibiting the breakdown of another potent endocannabinoid, anandamide[187] and via reduction of mast cell degranulation.[198] Although double-blind RCTs evaluating topical cannabinoids are not available, a multicenter prospective cohort study of 2456 patients reported that PEA 0.3% cream improved pruritus as well as other symptoms, including lichenification, excoriation, scaling, and erythema, in mild-to-moderate AD patients.[36] Daily use of PEA cream was associated with a 45.6% reduction in VAS score for itch 6 days after beginning treatment and with a 60% decrease after 6 weeks. In this study and in the author's experience, PEA creams are tolerated well with limited side effect, including occasional burning, itch, or mild erythema, usually limited to 1 to 2 applications[36] (unpublished observations).

Topical coal tar

Although the precise mechanism of action is unclear, topical formulations of crude and refined coal tar have been used for decades to treat inflammatory skin conditions, including AD.[199] Few studies evaluate the anti-inflammatory and antipruritic effects of coal tar in conditions other than psoriasis[199]; however 1 study demonstrated improvement in AD severity and itch in 18 subjects with mild to moderate AD after treatment with crude coal tar in a zinc paste at least 2 times to 3 times weekly.[200] An open-label comparative study found that a purified coal tar cream was as effective at reducing eczema and pruritus as 1% hydrocortisone cream.[201] Goeckerman therapy, which combines the use of crude coal tar and phototherapy, has also been used for decades to effectively reduce itch and inflammation in atopic patients with severe involvement.[38] Because it is well tolerated, safe, and cost-effective, coal tar has been suggested as a helpful, second-line, or adjunctive agent for AD management.[38,39]

Systemic Neuromodulators

Antiepileptics

Gabapentin and its prodrug pregabalin, analogs of the inhibitory neurotransmitter γ-aminobutyric acid, play a growing role in the management of neuropathic conditions including chronic pain and itch.[202–204] Their ability to reduce nociception is attributed to inhibition of voltage-gated sodium and calcium channels in dorsal root ganglia and spinal cord, respectively[205–207]; reduction in glutamate synthesis and release[203,207]; and decreased neural expression of SP and CGRP, both of which are increased in AD.[208]

Although the efficacy of neuroleptics in managing atopic itch has yet to be formally evaluated, numerous case reports, small case series, and placebo-controlled double-blind RCTs support a role for these agents in the management of other itchy dermatoses, including prurigo nodularis,[53,54] brachioradial pruritus,[209] notalgia paresthetica,[55] burn-related itch,[56,57] postherpetic itch,[210] cholestatic itch,[58] and uremic itch.[211,212] Although sedating effects can limit the rate of dose escalation during the day, gabapentin may be particularly helpful in reducing nocturnal pruritus and scratching in atopic patients. Due to myriad potential side effects, including fatigue, dizziness, blurred vision, nausea, dry mouth, and weight gain, it is prudent to start therapy at low doses (100–300 mg at bedtime) and slowly titrate upwards as tolerated.

Antidepressants

Serotonin and norepinephrine antidepressants

Selective serotonin reuptake inhibitors (SSRIs) block the reuptake of serotonin into presynaptic terminals, thereby increasing the effective concentration of serotonin in synaptic clefts and indirectly modulating presynaptic and postsynaptic serotonin receptors. Serotonin has pleiotropic effects in the skin, reflecting the widespread distribution of serotonin receptors on different cutaneous cell types, including peripheral sensory nerves, keratinocytes, mast cells, lymphocytes, natural killer cells, and Langerhans cells, among others.[213–215] In animal models, activation of serotonin 7 receptors on peripheral nerves mediates acute and chronic itch signals.[216] SSRIs have shown promise in reducing AD-related itch and prurigo nodularis as well as psychogenic pruritus, polycythemia vera, and cholestatic and paraneoplastic pruritus.[59–64] In a prospective, open-label trial comparing 2 SSRIs, both paroxetine and fluvoxamine decreased itch severity by approximal 50% in patients with chronic itch, including the subset of patients with AD.[59] Potential side effects of SSRIs include insomnia, weight loss, nausea, fatigue, and changes in sexual libido or function.

Mirtazapine, a serotonin and norepinephrine antidepressant, has been reported to reduce pruritus in AD as well as other chronic pruritic dermatoses.[65–67,159] Mirtazapine also exerts anxiolytic and antihistamine effects and the resultant sedative properties may well contribute to its antipruritic actions.[217] Although mirtazapine tends to exhibit fewer anticholinergic effects than SSRIs, users face greater challenges with sedation and weight gain. With all the medications in these classes, it is critical to taper patients off therapy slowly to avoid systemic rebound effects.

Aprepitant Aprepitant is an FDA-approved anti-emetic drug that inhibits the effects of SP on neurokinin-1 receptors in the central and peripheral nervous systems, including cutaneous nerve endings.[218,219] Although aprepitant has been reported effective in reducing itch in patients with prurigo nodularis[219] and in Sézary syndrome[220] in Europe, reports of its use elsewhere have failed to demonstrate improvement in itch in these conditions and it is has not yet been formally evaluated in AD.

Opioid modulators Opioids modulate the perception of pain and itch, exerting diverse actions, depending on the receptor activated (MORs, KORs, and δ-opioid receptors) and the site of action within the central and peripheral nervous systems.[221–223] Naltrexone and nalmefene, MOR antagonists, have been evaluated in the management of AD-related pruritus with promising results.[68] One double-blind RCT in AD and urticarial patients demonstrated that nalmefene significantly reduced or completely eliminated itch compared with placebo.[224] Several double-blind RCTs and open-label prospective trials demonstrate that naltrexone effectively reduces itch severity in atopic patients, in some cases within 2 weeks.[69,70] Moreover, oral naltrexone was found to reduce acute itch and alloknesis in AD patients.[71] Although a few studies failed to show improvement in atopic itch,[72] the current evidence generally supports the use of MOR antagonists as second-line or adjunctive agents in managing AD-related pruritus. MOR antagonists frequently trigger dose-dependent side effects, including dizziness, fatigue, gastrointestinal upset, or cramping.[68] To limit these effects, initiation of therapy with this class of medications should start with low doses (eg, nalmefene, 10 mg daily, and naltrexone, 25 mg daily) with a slow titration up over the course of weeks.[225]

Animal and human studies suggest that opioid activity in the periphery and spinal cord are critical modulators of itch transmission pathways and that an imbalance in endogenous μ-opioid and κ-opioid activity may result in certain types of chronic itch.[226–228] Consistent with these observations, nalfurafine, a selective KOR agonist, is approved to treat uremic itch in Japan, but has not been formally tested in AD.[229,230] Butorphanol, a combined MOR antagonist and KOR agonist, has been reported to benefit patients with intractable itch in the setting of primary biliary cirrhosis, paraneoplastic itch, and senile pruritus.[226] In addition to potential peripheral and spinal antagonism of itch pathways, recent functional neuroimaging studies found that butorphanol caused bilateral deactivation of neural structures involved in processing cowhage-induced itch (eg, claustrum, insula, and putamen) and was associated with altered cerebral perfusion activity in the midbrain, thalamus, S1, insula, and cerebellum.[231] Thus, butorphanol may be useful in reducing spinal and cortical processing of incoming itch signals, making it an attractive candidate for itch management for AD patients. Formal randomized controlled trials are still needed to evaluate this possibility.

ALTERNATIVE THERAPIES

Although complementary and alternative therapies (CATs) are becoming increasingly used in the management of chronic skin diseases, such as AD, few high-quality studies address their efficacy. A recent comprehensive meta-analysis of RCTs of CATs demonstrated efficacy of acupuncture and acupressure, hypnosis, massage, biofeedback, balneotherapy, herbal preparations, and oral evening primrose oil (EPO).[232] The evidence supporting the use of these CATs with respect to atopic itch is summarized.

Acupuncture and Acupressure

Acupuncture and acupressure are traditional practices of Chinese medicine in which specific points of the body are stimulated via the insertion of thin needles through or by applying direct pressure to skin, respectively. A systematic review of 70 RCTs of CATs for AD supports the use of acupuncture and acupressure as adjunctive measures in AD management.[232] Acupuncture reduces histamine and allergen-induced itch in healthy volunteers[233–236] and AD patients.[237] In a recent double-blind, placebo-controlled, crossover RCT, both verum acupuncture and cetirizine, reduced type 1 hypersensitivity-induced itch in AD patients.[238] In a randomized trial comparing standard care with or without acupressure in 15 AD patients, those receiving acupressure reported a significant decrease in itch VAS scores compared with subjects receiving standard care alone.[239] Functional MRI in AD patients showed that acupuncture produced a greater reduction in activation of central itch centers in response to an allergen, compared with oral antihistamines or placebo.[240] These and other studies provide reasonable support for the use of acupuncture to reduce AD-related itch.

Stress Reduction

Stress reduction techniques, such as habit reversal training (eg, learning to clench your fists instead of scratching in response to itch) and cognitive behavior therapy (CBT), have been reported to reduce the frequency and severity of itch in several types of dermatoses.[241-243] Atopic patients who took part in a stress relief program consisting of CBT, autogenic or self-suggestion relaxation therapy, or combined education and CBT experienced significantly less itch and scratched less than patients who received standard skin care alone.[244] Similarly, 20 minutes of daily massage therapy in addition to standard therapy has also been shown to significantly reduce itch severity in AD patients compared with those receiving standard therapy alone.[245] According to one report, a combination of stress-management psychotherapy, relaxation techniques, and habit reversal training provides the most effective strategy to combat itch in AD.[241]

Herbal Supplements and Botanic Oils

A growing number of AD patients supplement their standard skin care regimens with herbal remedies to help manage itch, including licorice root St. John's wort, Zemaphyte (a traditional Chinese mixture of 10 plant extracts), chamomile, and fern extracts.[232,246,247] A handful of RCTs evaluating various Chinese herbal therapy mixtures has demonstrated decreased itch, improved sleep quality, and reduced AD severity over time compared with placebo.[248,249] Commonly reported adverse effects of herbal mixtures include dizziness, nausea, dyspepsia, mild abdominal distention or pain, and headache.[250]

Several topical oils have shown beneficial in managing mild to moderate AD. Virgin coconut and olive oils are known to diminish colonization of S aureus in atopic patients; however, the former was proved superior to virgin olive oil in controlling AD severity and colonization[20] and similar to mineral oil in reducing clinical severity and TEWL.[251] EPO and borage oil contain high levels of γ-linoleic acid and omega-6 fatty acids, which may indirectly promote barrier repair and reduce cutaneous inflammation.[252] When applied topically, both EPO and borage oil reduce eczema severity and itch,[253,254] although no clear benefit has been shown for oral supplementation with these agents.[255]

Recommendations and Therapeutic Ladder

Given the numerous and diverse factors that contribute to AD, a multifaceted approach to disease management is key. Central to this goal is controlling itch symptoms and the vicious cycles triggered by scratching. In general, all patients with AD should be educated on the benefits of stress management, adequate sleep, and barrier protection from irritants and pathogens, because such interventions form the cornerstone of managing itch and inflammation in AD. Care providers should elicit and discuss alternative therapies that patients are incorporating into their therapeutic regimen and, if possible, make encourage or suggest complementary strategies, such as acupuncture, relaxation techniques, and meditation.

For active disease, the judicious use of topical or systemic immunosuppressive agents and/or phototherapy is recommended. Neuromodulators may benefit AD patients in managing itch regardless of disease severity. Based on the data discussed previously and the author's experience, localized or mild disease is often well controlled with topical naltrexone, PEA-containing creams (whether commercially available or compounded), compounded 3% to 5% urea plus topical anesthetics, or evening dosing of oral gabapentin (300–600 mg daily) or sedating antihistamines. As itch severity progresses, combined topical and oral therapy with SSRIs (dosed during the day), mirtazapine (dosed at bedtime), and neuroleptics (dosed multiple times throughout the day [eg, gabapentin 600 mg 3 times daily]) may be warranted. When systemic agents are used, it is the author's practice to initiate low-dose therapy at night to assess tolerance and mitigate nocturnal itch before adding daytime doses. As the use of neural-targeted therapies continues to grow, more rigorous evaluation of their ability to control AD-related itch and disease burden, as well as the putative pathways involved, will be required.

REFERENCES

1. Drucker AM, Wang AR, Li WQ, et al. The Burden of Atopic Dermatitis: Summary of a Report for the National Eczema Association. J Invest Dermatol 2017; 137(1):26–30.
2. Chuquilin M, Alghalith Y, Fernandez KH. Neurocutaneous disease: cutaneous neuroanatomy and mechanisms of itch and pain. J Am Acad Dermatol 2016;74(2):197–212.
3. Ross SE, Mardinly AR, McCord AE, et al. Loss of inhibitory interneurons in the dorsal spinal cord and elevated itch in Bhlhb5 mutant mice. Neuron 2010;65(6):886–98.
4. Ross SE, Hachisuka J, Todd AJ. Spinal microcircuits and the regulation of itch. In: Carstens E, Akiyama T, editors. Itch: mechanisms and treatment. Boca Raton (FL): CRC Press/Taylor & Francis; 2014. Chapter 20.
5. Ikoma A, Fartasch M, Heyer G, et al. Painful stimuli evoke itch in patients with chronic pruritus: central sensitization for itch. Neurology 2004;62(2):212–7.
6. Pincelli C, Fantini F, Massimi P, et al. Neuropeptides in skin from patients with atopic dermatitis: an

immunohistochemical study. Br J Dermatol 1990; 122(6):745–50.

7. Anand P, Springall DR, Blank MA, et al. Neuropeptides in skin disease: increased VIP in eczema and psoriasis but not axillary hyperhidrosis. Br J Dermatol 1991;124(6):547–9.

8. Mollanazar NK, Smith PK, Yosipovitch G. Mediators of chronic pruritus in atopic dermatitis: getting the itch out? Clin Rev Allergy Immunol 2015;51(3):263–92.

9. Steinhoff M, Neisius U, Ikoma A, et al. Proteinase-activated receptor-2 mediates itch: a novel pathway for pruritus in human skin. J Neurosci 2003;23(15):6176–80.

10. Akiyama T, Merrill AW, Carstens MI, et al. Activation of superficial dorsal horn neurons in the mouse by a PAR-2 agonist and 5-HT: potential role in itch. J Neurosci 2009;29(20):6691–9.

11. Andoh T, Kuraishi Y. Intradermal leukotriene B4, but not prostaglandin E2, induces itch-associated responses in mice. Eur J Pharmacol 1998;353(1):93–6.

12. Ikoma A, Steinhoff M, Ständer S, et al. The neurobiology of itch. Nat Rev Neurosci 2006;7(7):535–47.

13. Heyer G, Vogelgsang M, Hornstein OP. Acetylcholine is an inducer of itching in patients with atopic eczema. J Dermatol 1997;24(10):621–5.

14. Hosogi M, Schmelz M, Miyachi Y, et al. Bradykinin is a potent pruritogen in atopic dermatitis: a switch from pain to itch. Pain 2006;126(1–3):16–23.

15. Cevikbas F, Wang X, Akiyama T, et al. A sensory neuron-expressed IL-31 receptor mediates T helper cell-dependent itch: involvement of TRPV1 and TRPA1. J Allergy Clin Immunol 2014;133:448–60.

16. Kashem SW, Riedl MS, Yao C, et al. Nociceptive sensory fibers drive interleukin-23 production from CD301b+ dermal dendritic cells and drive protective cutaneous immunity. Immunity 2015; 43(3):515–26.

17. Chiu IM, Heesters BA, Ghasemlou N, et al. Bacteria activate sensory neurons that modulate pain and inflammation. Nature 2013;501(7465):52–7.

18. Peris K, Valeri P, Altobelli E, et al. Efficacy evaluation of an oil-in-water emulsion (Dermoflan) in atopic dermatitis. Acta Derm Venereol 2002;82(6):465–6.

19. Korting HC, Schollmann C, Cholcha W, et al, Collaborative Study Group. Efficacy and tolerability of pale sulfonated shale oil cream 4% in the treatment of mild to moderate atopic eczema in children: a multicentre, randomized vehicle-controlled trial. J Eur Acad Dermatol Venereol 2010;24(10):1176–82.

20. Verallo-Rowell VM, Dillague KM, Syah-Tjundawan BS. Novel antibacterial and emollient effects of coconut and virgin olive oils in adult atopic dermatitis. Dermatitis 2008;19(6):308–15.

21. Matsumoto T, Yuasa H, Kai R, et al. Skin capacitance in normal and atopic infants, and effects of moisturizers on atopic skin. J Dermatol 2007; 34(7):447–50.

22. Breternitz M, Kowatzki D, Langenauer M, et al. Placebo-controlled, double-blind, randomized, prospective study of a glycerol-based emollient on eczematous skin in atopic dermatitis: biophysical and clinical evaluation. Skin Pharmacol Physiol 2008;21(1):39–45.

23. Grimalt R, Mengeaud V, Cambazard F, et al. The steroid-sparing effect of an emollient therapy in infants with atopic dermatitis: a randomized controlled study. Dermatology 2007;214(1):61–7.

24. Chamlin SL, McCalmont TH, Cunningham BB, et al. Cutaneous manifestations of hyper-IgE syndrome in infants and children. J Pediatr 2002;141(4): 572–5.

25. Kircik LH, Del Rosso JQ, Aversa D. Evaluating Clinical Use of a Ceramide-dominant, Physiologic Lipid-based Topical Emulsion for Atopic Dermatitis. J Clin Aesthet Dermatol 2011;4(3):34–40.

26. Hoare C, Li Wan Po A, Williams H. Systematic review of treatments for atopic eczema. Health Technol Assess 2000;4(37):1–191.

27. Boguniewicz M, Fiedler VC, Raimer S, et al. A randomized, vehicle-controlled trial of tacrolimus ointment for treatment of atopic dermatitis in children. Pediatric Tacrolimus Study Group. J Allergy Clin Immunol 1998;102(4 Pt 1):637–44.

28. Paller A, Eichenfield LF, Leung DY, et al. A 12-week study of tacrolimus ointment for the treatment of atopic dermatitis in pediatric patients. J Am Acad Dermatol 2001;44(1 Suppl):S47–57.

29. Schachner LA, Lamerson C, Sheehan MP, et al, US Tacrolimus Ointment Study Group. Tacrolimus ointment 0.03% is safe and effective for the treatment of mild to moderate atopic dermatitis in pediatric patients: results from a randomized, double-blind, vehicle-controlled study. Pediatrics 2005;116(3): e334–342.

30. Drake LA, Fallon JD, Sober A. Relief of pruritus in patients with atopic dermatitis after treatment with topical doxepin cream. The Doxepin Study Group. J Am Acad Dermatol 1994;31(4):613–6.

31. Bath-Hextall FJ, Birnie AJ, Ravenscroft JC, et al. Interventions to reduce Staphylococcus aureus in the management of atopic eczema: an updated Cochrane review. Br J Dermatol 2010;163(1):12–26.

32. Freeman CW. A new topical remedy useful in the management of pruritus. J Natl Med Assoc 1961; 53:151–3.

33. Hawro T, Fluhr JW, Mengeaud V, et al. Polidocanol inhibits cowhage - but not histamine-induced itch in humans. Exp Dermatol 2014;23(12):922–3.

34. Freitag G, Hoppner T. Results of a postmarketing drug monitoring survey with a polidocanol-urea preparation for dry, itching skin. Curr Med Res Opin 1997;13(9):529–37.

35. Riser RL, Kowcz A, Schoelermann A, et al. Tolerance profile and efficacy of a menthol-containing

itch relief spray in children and atopics. Br. J. Derm 2003;149:83.

36. Eberlein B, Eicke C, Reinhardt HW, et al. Adjuvant treatment of atopic eczema: assessment of an emollient containing N-palmitoylethanolamine (ATOPA study). J Eur Acad Dermatol Venereol 2008;22(1):73–82.

37. Bigliardi PL, Stammer H, Jost G, et al. Treatment of pruritus with topically applied opiate receptor antagonist. J Am Acad Dermatol 2007;56(6):979–88.

38. Hong J, Buddenkotte J, Berger TG, et al. Management of itch in atopic dermatitis. Semin Cutan Med Surg 2011;30(2):71–86.

39. Roelofzen JH, Aben KK, Oldenhof UT, et al. No increased risk of cancer after coal tar treatment in patients with psoriasis or eczema. J Invest Dermatol 2010;130(4):953–61.

40. Kelsay K. Management of sleep disturbance associated with atopic dermatitis. J Allergy Clin Immunol 2006;118(1):198–201.

41. Klein PA, Clark RA. An evidence-based review of the efficacy of antihistamines in relieving pruritus in atopic dermatitis. Arch Dermatol 1999;135(12):1522–5.

42. Kawashima M, Tango T, Noguchi T, et al. Addition of fexofenadine to a topical corticosteroid reduces the pruritus associated with atopic dermatitis in a 1-week randomized, multicentre, double-blind, placebo-controlled, parallel-group study. Br J Dermatol 2003;148(6):1212–21.

43. Schmitt J, Schmitt N, Meurer M. Cyclosporin in the treatment of patients with atopic eczema - a systematic review and meta-analysis. J Eur Acad Dermatol Venereol 2007;21(5):606–19.

44. Harper JI, Ahmed I, Barclay G, et al. Cyclosporin for severe childhood atopic dermatitis: short course versus continuous therapy. Br J Dermatol 2000;142(1):52–8.

45. Pacor ML, Di Lorenzo G, Martinelli N, et al. Comparing tacrolimus ointment and oral cyclosporine in adult patients affected by atopic dermatitis: a randomized study. Clin Exp Allergy 2004;34(4):639–45.

46. Czech W, Brautigam M, Weidinger G, et al. A body-weight-independent dosing regimen of cyclosporine microemulsion is effective in severe atopic dermatitis and improves the quality of life. J Am Acad Dermatol 2000;42(4):653–9.

47. Schram ME, Roekevisch E, Leeflang MM, et al. A randomized trial of methotrexate versus azathioprine for severe atopic eczema. J Allergy Clin Immunol 2011;128(2):353–9.

48. Berth-Jones J, Takwale A, Tan E, et al. Azathioprine in severe adult atopic dermatitis: a double-blind, placebo-controlled, crossover trial. Br J Dermatol 2002;147(2):324–30.

49. Neuber K, Schwartz I, Itschert G, et al. Treatment of atopic eczema with oral mycophenolate mofetil. Br J Dermatol 2000;143(2):385–91.

50. Jackson JM, Fowler JF Jr, Callen JP, et al. Mycophenolate mofetil for the treatment of chronic dermatitis: an open-label study of 16 patients. J Drugs Dermatol 2010;9(4):356–62.

51. Haeck IM, Knol MJ, Ten Berge O, et al. Enteric-coated mycophenolate sodium versus cyclosporin A as long-term treatment in adult patients with severe atopic dermatitis: a randomized controlled trial. J Am Acad Dermatol 2011;64(6):1074–84.

52. Weatherhead SC, Wahie S, Reynolds NJ, et al. An open-label, dose-ranging study of methotrexate for moderate-to-severe adult atopic eczema. Br J Dermatol 2007;156(2):346–51.

53. Mazza M, Guerriero G, Marano G, et al. Treatment of prurigo nodularis with pregabalin. J Clin Pharm Ther 2013;38(1):16–8.

54. Fostini AC, Girolomoni G, Tessari G. Prurigo nodularis: an update on etiopathogenesis and therapy. J Dermatolog Treat 2013;24(6):458–62.

55. Loosemore MP, Bordeaux JS, Bernhard JD. Gabapentin treatment for notalgia paresthetica, a common isolated peripheral sensory neuropathy. J Eur Acad Dermatol Venereol 2007;21(10):1440–1.

56. Goutos I, Clarke M, Upson C, et al. Review of therapeutic agents for burns pruritus and protocols for management in adult and paediatric patients using the GRADE classification. Indian J Plast Surg 2010;43(Suppl):S51–62.

57. Ahuja RB, Gupta GK. A four arm, double blind, randomized and placebo controlled study of pregabalin in the management of post-burn pruritus. Burns 2013;39(1):24–9.

58. Bergasa NV, McGee M, Ginsburg IH, et al. Gabapentin in patients with the pruritus of cholestasis: a double-blind, randomized, placebo-controlled trial. Hepatology 2006;44(5):1317–23.

59. Stander S, Bockenholt B, Schurmeyer-Horst F, et al. Treatment of chronic pruritus with the selective serotonin re-uptake inhibitors paroxetine and fluvoxamine: results of an open-labelled, two-arm proof-of-concept study. Acta Derm Venereol 2009;89(1):45–51.

60. Tefferi A, Fonseca R. Selective serotonin reuptake inhibitors are effective in the treatment of polycythemia vera-associated pruritus. Blood 2002;99(7):2627.

61. Zylicz Z, Smits C, Krajnik M. Paroxetine for pruritus in advanced cancer. J Pain Symptom Manage 1998;16(2):121–4.

62. Biondi M, Arcangeli T, Petrucci RM. Paroxetine in a case of psychogenic pruritus and neurotic excoriations. Psychother Psychosom 2000;69(3):165–6.

63. Zylicz Z, Krajnik M, Sorge AA, et al. Paroxetine in the treatment of severe non-dermatological

pruritus: a randomized, controlled trial. J Pain Symptom Manage 2003;26(6):1105–12.

64. Mayo MJ, Handem I, Saldana S, et al. Sertraline as a first-line treatment for cholestatic pruritus. Hepatology 2007;45(3):666–74.

65. Davis MP, Frandsen JL, Walsh D, et al. Mirtazapine for pruritus. J Pain Symptom Manage 2003;25(3): 288–91.

66. Hundley JL, Yosipovitch G. Mirtazapine for reducing nocturnal itch in patients with chronic pruritus: a pilot study. J Am Acad Dermatol 2004;50(6):889–91.

67. Demierre MF, Taverna J. Mirtazapine and gabapentin for reducing pruritus in cutaneous T-cell lymphoma. J Am Acad Dermatol 2006;55(3):543–4.

68. Phan NQ, Bernhard JD, Luger TA, et al. Antipruritic treatment with systemic mu-opioid receptor antagonists: a review. J Am Acad Dermatol 2010;63(4): 680–8.

69. Metze D, Reimann S, Beissert S, et al. Efficacy and safety of naltrexone, an oral opiate receptor antagonist, in the treatment of pruritus in internal and dermatological diseases. J Am Acad Dermatol 1999;41(4):533–9.

70. Malekzad F, Arbabi M, Mohtasham N, et al. Efficacy of oral naltrexone on pruritus in atopic eczema: a double-blind, placebo-controlled study. J Eur Acad Dermatol Venereol 2009;23(8):948–50.

71. Heyer G, Groene D, Martus P. Efficacy of naltrexone on acetylcholine-induced alloknesis in atopic eczema. Exp Dermatol 2002;11(5):448–55.

72. Burch JR, Harrison PV. Opiates, sleep and itch. Clin Exp Dermatol 1988;13(6):418–9.

73. Saeki H, Furue M, Furukawa F, et al, Committee for Guidelines for the Management of Atopic Dermatitis of Japanese Dermatological Association. Guidelines for management of atopic dermatitis. J Dermatol 2009;36(10):563–77.

74. Ellis C, Luger T, Abeck D, et al, ICCAD II Faculty. International consensus conference on atopic dermatitis II (ICCAD II): clinical update and current treatment strategies. Br J Dermatol 2003; 148(Suppl 63):3–10.

75. Eichenfield LF, Hanifin JM, Luger TA, et al. Consensus conference on pediatric atopic dermatitis. J Am Acad Dermatol 2003;49(6):1088–95.

76. Tadicherla S, Ross K, Shenefelt PD, et al. Topical corticosteroids in dermatology. J Drugs Dermatol 2009;8(12):1093–105.

77. Hanifin JM. Atopic dermatitis: broadening the perspective. J Am Acad Dermatol 2004;51(1 Suppl):S23–4.

78. Wahlgren CF, Hagermark O, Bergstrom R, et al. Evaluation of a new method of assessing pruritus and antipruritic drugs. Skin Pharmacol 1988;1(1): 3–13.

79. Maloney JM, Morman MR, Stewart DM, et al. Clobetasol propionate emollient 0.05% in the treatment of atopic dermatitis. Int J Dermatol 1998;37(2):142–4.

80. Sher LG, Chang J, Patel IB, et al. Relieving the pruritus of atopic dermatitis: a meta-analysis. Acta Derm Venereol 2012;92(5):455–61.

81. Kaplan RJ, Daman L, Rosenberg EW, et al. Topical use of caffeine with hydrocortisone in the treatment of atopic dermatitis. Arch Dermatol 1978;114(1): 60–2.

82. Roth HL, Brown EP. Hydrocortisone valerate. Double-blind comparison with two other topical steroids. Cutis 1978;21(5):695–8.

83. Sefton J, Kyriakopoulos AA. Comparative efficacy of hydrocortisone valerate 0.2 percent ointment in the treatment of atopic dermatitis. Cutis 1983; 32(1):89–91, 94.

84. Lassus A. Clinical comparison of alclometasone dipropionate cream 0.05% with hydrocortisone butyrate cream 0.1% in the treatment of atopic dermatitis in children. J Int Med Res 1983;11(5): 315–9.

85. Lassus A. Alclometasone dipropionate cream 0.05% versus clobetasone butyrate cream 0.05%. A controlled clinical comparison in the treatment of atopic dermatitis in children. Int J Dermatol 1984;23(8):565–6.

86. Bornhovd EC, Burgdorf WH, Wollenberg A. Immunomodulatory macrolactams for topical treatment of inflammatory skin diseases. Curr Opin Investig Drugs 2002;3(5):708–12.

87. Stander S, Schurmeyer-Horst F, Luger TA, et al. Treatment of pruritic diseases with topical calcineurin inhibitors. Ther Clin Risk Manag 2006;2(2):213–8.

88. Senba E, Katanosaka K, Yajima H, et al. The immunosuppressant FK506 activates capsaicin- and bradykinin-sensitive DRG neurons and cutaneous C-fibers. Neurosci Res 2004;50(3):257–62.

89. Kaufmann R, Bieber T, Helgesen AL, et al, Multicentre Investigator Group. Onset of pruritus relief with pimecrolimus cream 1% in adult patients with atopic dermatitis: a randomized trial. Allergy 2006;61(3):375–81.

90. Eichenfield LF, Lucky AW, Boguniewicz M, et al. Safety and efficacy of pimecrolimus (ASM 981) cream 1% in the treatment of mild and moderate atopic dermatitis in children and adolescents. J Am Acad Dermatol 2002;46(4):495–504.

91. Langley RG, Eichenfield LF, Lucky AW, et al. Sustained efficacy and safety of pimecrolimus cream 1% when used long-term (up to 26 weeks) to treat children with atopic dermatitis. Pediatr Dermatol 2008;25(3):301–7.

92. Paller AS, Lebwohl M, Fleischer AB Jr, et al, US/Canada Tacrolimus Ointment Study Group. Tacrolimus ointment is more effective than pimecrolimus cream with a similar safety profile in the treatment of atopic dermatitis: results from 3 randomized,

comparative studies. J Am Acad Dermatol 2005; 52(5):810–22.

93. McCollum AD, Paik A, Eichenfield LF. The safety and efficacy of tacrolimus ointment in pediatric patients with atopic dermatitis. Pediatr Dermatol 2010;27(5):425–36.

94. Paller AS, Eichenfield LF, Kirsner RS, et al, US Tacrolimus Ointment Study Group. Three times weekly tacrolimus ointment reduces relapse in stabilized atopic dermatitis: a new paradigm for use. Pediatrics 2008;122(6):e1210–1218.

95. Arellano FM, Wentworth CE, Arana A, et al. Risk of lymphoma following exposure to calcineurin inhibitors and topical steroids in patients with atopic dermatitis. J Invest Dermatol 2007;127(4):808–16.

96. Ohtsuki M, OH, Santos V, et al. Safety profiles of two large cohort studies of tacrolimus ointment for the treatment of atopic dermatitis: a prospective pediatric longitudinal evaluation study (APPLES) and Japanese long-term safety study (J-LSS). Paper presented at the Proceedings of the 22nd World Congress of Dermatology Meeting. Seoul, Korea, May 24, 2011.

97. Kothary N. Update on post-marketing AERS cases of pediatric malignancies reports with topical pimecrolimus and tacrolimus use. Paper presented at the Food and Drug Administration Pediatric Advisory Committee. Silver Springs (MD), May 16, 2011.

98. AO1 Segal, Ellis AK, Kim HL. CSACI position statement: safety of topical calcineurin inhibitors in the management of atopic dermatitis in children and adults. Allergy Asthma Clin Immunol 2013;9(1):24.

99. Allen B. A multicenter double-blind lacebo controlled crossover to assess the efficacy and safety of cyclosporin A in adult patients with severe refractory atopic dermatitis. Paper presented at the Second Congress of the European Academy of Dermatology and Venereology. Athens (Greece), October 12, 1991.

100. Darsow U, Scharein E, Bromm B, et al. Skin testing of the pruritogenic activity of histamine and cytokines (interleukin-2 and tumour necrosis factor-alpha) at the dermal-epidermal junction. Br J Dermatol 1997;137(3):415–7.

101. Wahlgren CF, Scheynius A, Hagermark O. Antipruritic effect of oral cyclosporin A in atopic dermatitis. Acta Derm Venereol 1990;70(4):323–9.

102. Schmitt J, Schakel K, Schmitt N, et al. Systemic treatment of severe atopic eczema: a systematic review. Acta Derm Venereol 2007;87(2):100–11.

103. Madan V, Griffiths CE. Systemic ciclosporin and tacrolimus in dermatology. Dermatol Ther 2007; 20(4):239–50.

104. Roekevisch E, Spuls PI, Kuester D, et al. Efficacy and safety of systemic treatments for moderate-to-severe atopic dermatitis: a systematic review. J Allergy Clin Immunol 2014;133(2):429–38.

105. Meggitt SJ, Gray JC, Reynolds NJ. Azathioprine dosed by thiopurine methyltransferase activity for moderate-to-severe atopic eczema: a double-blind, randomised controlled trial. Lancet 2006; 367(9513):839–46.

106. Yarbrough KB, Neuhaus KJ, Simpson EL. The effects of treatment on itch in atopic dermatitis. Dermatol Ther 2013;26(2):110–9.

107. Beck LA, Thaci D, Hamilton JD, et al. Dupilumab treatment in adults with moderate-to-severe atopic dermatitis. N Engl J Med 2014;371(2):130–9.

108. Thaci D, Simpson EL, Beck LA, et al. Efficacy and safety of dupilumab in adults with moderate-to-severe atopic dermatitis inadequately controlled by topical treatments: a randomised, placebo-controlled, dose-ranging phase 2b trial. Lancet 2016;387(10013):40–52.

109. Zink A, Gensbaur A, Zirbs M, et al. Targeting IgE in Severe atopic dermatitis with a combination of immunoadsorption and omalizumab. Acta Derm Venereol 2016;96(1):72–6.

110. Heil PM, Maurer D, Klein B, et al. Omalizumab therapy in atopic dermatitis: depletion of IgE does not improve the clinical course - a randomized, placebo-controlled and double blind pilot study. J Dtsch Dermatol Ges 2010;8(12):990–8.

111. Hotze M, Baurecht H, Rodríguez E, et al. Increased efficacy of omalizumab in atopic dermatitis patients with wild-type filaggrin status and higher serum levels of phosphatidylcholines. Allergy 2014; 69(1):132–5.

112. Rivard J, Lim HW. Ultraviolet phototherapy for pruritus. Dermatol Ther 2005;18(4):344–54.

113. Piletta PA, Wirth S, Hommel L, et al. Circulating skin-homing T cells in atopic dermatitis. Selective up-regulation of HLA-DR, interleukin-2R, and CD30 and decrease after combined UV-A and UV-B phototherapy. Arch Dermatol 1996;132(10):1171–6.

114. Grabbe J, Welker P, Humke S, et al. High-dose ultraviolet A1 (UVA1), but not UVA/UVB therapy, decreases IgE-binding cells in lesional skin of patients with atopic eczema. J Invest Dermatol 1996;107(3):419–22.

115. Wallengren J, Sundler F. Phototherapy reduces the number of epidermal and CGRP-positive dermal nerve fibres. Acta Derm Venereol 2004; 84(2):111–5.

116. Jekler J, Larko O. UVB phototherapy of atopic dermatitis. Br J Dermatol 1988;119(6):697–705.

117. Clayton TH, Clark SM, Turner D, et al. The treatment of severe atopic dermatitis in childhood with narrowband ultraviolet B phototherapy. Clin Exp Dermatol 2007;32(1):28–33.

118. Jekler J, Larko O. Combined UVA-UVB versus UVB phototherapy for atopic dermatitis: a paired-comparison study. J Am Acad Dermatol 1990; 22(1):49–53.

119. von Kobyletzki G, Pieck C, Hoffmann K, et al. Medium-dose UVA1 cold-light phototherapy in the treatment of severe atopic dermatitis. J Am Acad Dermatol 1999;41(6):931–7.

120. Sheehan MP, Atherton DJ, Norris P, et al. Oral psoralen photochemotherapy in severe childhood atopic eczema: an update. Br J Dermatol 1993; 129(4):431–6.

121. Der-Petrossian M, Seeber A, Honigsmann H, et al. Half-side comparison study on the efficacy of 8-methoxypsoralen bath-PUVA versus narrowband ultraviolet B phototherapy in patients with severe chronic atopic dermatitis. Br J Dermatol 2000; 142(1):39–43.

122. Reynolds NJ, Franklin V, Gray JC, et al. Narrowband ultraviolet B and broad-band ultraviolet A phototherapy in adult atopic eczema: a randomised controlled trial. Lancet 2001;357(9273): 2012–6.

123. Uetsu N, Horio T. Treatment of persistent severe atopic dermatitis in 113 Japanese patients with oral psoralen photo-chemotherapy. J Dermatol 2003;30(6):450–7.

124. Archier E, Devaux S, Castela E, et al. Carcinogenic risks of psoralen UV-A therapy and narrowband UV-B therapy in chronic plaque psoriasis: a systematic literature review. J Eur Acad Dermatol Venereol 2012;(Suppl 3):22–31.

125. Yamamoto A, Serizawa S, Ito M, et al. Stratum corneum lipid abnormalities in atopic dermatitis. Arch Dermatol Res 1991;283(4):219–23.

126. Weidinger S, O'Sullivan M, Illig T, et al. Filaggrin mutations, atopic eczema, hay fever, and asthma in children. J Allergy Clin Immunol 2008;121(5):1203–9.e1.

127. Werner Y, Lindberg M. Transepidermal water loss in dry and clinically normal skin in patients with atopic dermatitis. Acta Derm Venereol 1985;65(2):102–5.

128. Elmariah SB, Lerner EA. Topical therapies for pruritus. Semin Cutan Med Surg 2011;30(2):118–26.

129. Vilaplana J, Coll J, Trullas C, et al. Clinical and non-invasive evaluation of 12% ammonium lactate emulsion for the treatment of dry skin in atopic and non-atopic subjects. Acta Derm Venereol 1992;72(1):28–33.

130. Szczepanowska J, Reich A, Szepietowski JC. Emollients improve treatment results with topical corticosteroids in childhood atopic dermatitis: a randomized comparative study. Pediatr Allergy Immunol 2008;19(7):614–8.

131. Kurtz ES, Wallo W. Colloidal oatmeal: history, chemistry and clinical properties. J Drugs Dermatol 2007;6(2):167–70.

132. Alexandrescu DT, Vaillant JG, Dasanu CA. Effect of treatment with a colloidal oatmeal lotion on the acneform eruption induced by epidermal growth factor receptor and multiple tyrosine-kinase inhibitors. Clin Exp Dermatol 2007;32(1):71–4.

133. Sur R, Nigam A, Grote D, et al. Avenanthramides, polyphenols from oats, exhibit anti-inflammatory and anti-itch activity. Arch Dermatol Res 2008; 300(10):569–74.

134. Fowler JF, Nebus J, Wallo W, et al. Colloidal oatmeal formulations as adjunct treatments in atopic dermatitis. J Drugs Dermatol 2012;11(7):804–7.

135. Grayson S, Elias PM. Isolation and lipid biochemical characterization of stratum corneum membrane complexes: implications for the cutaneous permeability barrier. J Invest Dermatol 1982;78(2):128–35.

136. Wertz PW, Downing DT. Ceramides of pig epidermis: structure determination. J Lipid Res 1983;24(6):759–65.

137. Di Nardo A, Wertz P, Giannetti A, et al. Ceramide and cholesterol composition of the skin of patients with atopic dermatitis. Acta Derm Venereol 1998; 78(1):27–30.

138. Imokawa G, Abe A, Jin K, et al. Decreased level of ceramides in stratum corneum of atopic dermatitis: an etiologic factor in atopic dry skin? J Invest Dermatol 1991;96(4):523–6.

139. Lynde CW, Andriessen A. A cohort study on a ceramide-containing cleanser and moisturizer used for atopic dermatitis. Cutis 2014;93(4):207–13.

140. Zettersten EM, Ghadially R, Feingold KR, et al. Optimal ratios of topical stratum corneum lipids improve barrier recovery in chronologically aged skin. J Am Acad Dermatol 1997;37(3 Pt 1):403–8.

141. Patrizi A, Capitanio B, Neri I, et al. A double-blind, randomized, vehicle-controlled clinical study to evaluate the efficacy and safety of MAS063DP (ATOPICLAIR) in the management of atopic dermatitis in paediatric patients. Pediatr Allergy Immunol 2008;19(7):619–25.

142. Abramovits W, Boguniewicz M, Adult Atopiclair Study G. A multicenter, randomized, vehicle-controlled clinical study to examine the efficacy and safety of MAS063DP (Atopiclair) in the management of mild to moderate atopic dermatitis in adults. J Drugs Dermatol 2006;5(3):236–44.

143. Bikowski J. Case studies assessing a new skin barrier repair cream for the treatment of atopic dermatitis. J Drugs Dermatol 2009;8(11):1037–41.

144. Simpson EL. Atopic dermatitis: a review of topical treatment options. Curr Med Res Opin 2010; 26(3):633–40.

145. Ali SM, Yosipovitch G. Skin pH: from basic science to basic skin care. Acta Derm Venereol 2013;93(3): 261–7.

146. Boguniewicz M, Sampson H, Leung SB, et al. Effects of cefuroxime axetil on Staphylococcus aureus colonization and superantigen production in atopic dermatitis. J Allergy Clin Immunol 2001; 108(4):651–2.

147. Bunikowski R, Mielke ME, Skarabis H, et al. Evidence for a disease-promoting effect of Staphylococcus

aureus-derived exotoxins in atopic dermatitis. J Allergy Clin Immunol 2000;105(4):814–9.

148. Zollner TM, Wichelhaus TA, Hartung A, et al. Colonization with superantigen-producing Staphylococcus aureus is associated with increased severity of atopic dermatitis. Clin Exp Allergy 2000;30(7):994–1000.

149. Wichmann K, Uter W, Weiss J, et al. Isolation of alpha-toxin-producing Staphylococcus aureus from the skin of highly sensitized adult patients with severe atopic dermatitis. Br J Dermatol 2009; 161(2):300–5.

150. Hauser C, Wuethrich B, Matter L, et al. Staphylococcus aureus skin colonization in atopic dermatitis patients. Dermatologica 1985;170(1):35–9.

151. Leyden JJ, Kligman AM. The case for steroid–antibiotic combinations. Br J Dermatol 1977;96(2): 179–87.

152. Birnie AJ, Bath-Hextall FJ, Ravenscroft JC, et al. Interventions to reduce Staphylococcus aureus in the management of atopic eczema. Cochrane Database Syst Rev 2008;(3):CD003871.

153. Huang JT, Abrams M, Tlougan B, et al. Treatment of Staphylococcus aureus colonization in atopic dermatitis decreases disease severity. Pediatrics 2009;123(5):e808–814.

154. Wong SM, Ng TG, Baba R. Efficacy and safety of sodium hypochlorite (bleach) baths in patients with moderate to severe atopic dermatitis in Malaysia. J Dermatol 2013;40(11):874–80.

155. Lewis T, Zotterman Y. Vascular reactions of the skin to injury: Part VIII. The resistance of the human skin to constant currents, in relation to injury and vascular response. J Physiol 1927;62(3):280–8.

156. Albrecht M, Dittrich AM. Expression and function of histamine and its receptors in atopic dermatitis. Mol Cell Pediatr 2015;2(1):16.

157. Epstein E, Pinski JB. A blind study. Arch Dermatol 1964;89:548–9.

158. Diepgen TL, Early Treatment of the Atopic Child Study, Group. Long-term treatment with cetirizine of infants with atopic dermatitis: a multi-country, double-blind, randomized, placebo-controlled trial (the ETAC trial) over 18 months. Pediatr Allergy Immunol 2002;13(4):278–86.

159. Hannuksela M, Kalimo K, Lammintausta K, et al. Dose ranging study: cetirizine in the treatment of atopic dermatitis in adults. Ann Allergy 1993; 70(2):127–33.

160. Richardson GS, Roehrs TA, Rosenthal L, et al. Tolerance to daytime sedative effects of H1 antihistamines. J Clin Psychopharmacol 2002;5: 511–5.

161. Shelley WB, Shelley ED, Talanin NY. Self-potentiating allergic contact dermatitis caused by doxepin hydrochloride cream. J Am Acad Dermatol 1996;34(1):143–4.

162. Greaves MW. Antihistamines in dermatology. Skin Pharmacol Physiol 2005;18(5):220–9.

163. Misery L. Atopic dermatitis and the nervous system. Clin Rev Allergy Immunol 2011;41(3):259–66.

164. Barry R, Rogers S. Brachioradial pruritus–an enigmatic entity. Clin Exp Dermatol 2004;29(6):637–8.

165. Knight TE, Hayashi T. Solar (brachioradial) pruritus–response to capsaicin cream. Int J Dermatol 1994;33(3):206–9.

166. Lysy J, Sistiery-Ittah M, Israelit Y, et al. Topical capsaicin–a novel and effective treatment for idiopathic intractable pruritus ani: a randomised, placebo controlled, crossover study. Gut 2003;52(9):1323–6.

167. Makhlough A, Ala S, Haj-Heydari Z, et al. Topical capsaicin therapy for uremic pruritus in patients on hemodialysis. Iran J Kidney Dis 2010;4(2):137–40.

168. Stander S, Luger T, Metze D. Treatment of prurigo nodularis with topical capsaicin. J Am Acad Dermatol 2001;44(3):471–8.

169. Lotti T, Teofoli P, Tsampau D. Treatment of aquagenic pruritus with topical capsaicin cream. J Am Acad Dermatol 1994;30(2 Pt 1):232–5.

170. Caterina MJ, Schumacher MA, Tominaga M, et al. The capsaicin receptor: a heat-activated ion channel in the pain pathway. Nature 1997;389(6653):816–24.

171. Dray A. Neuropharmacological mechanisms of capsaicin and related substances. Biochem Pharmacol 1992;44(4):611–5.

172. Zhang WY, Li Wan Po A. The effectiveness of topically applied capsaicin. A meta-analysis. Eur J Clin Pharmacol 1994;46(6):517–22.

173. Gooding SM, Canter PH, Coelho HF, et al. Systematic review of topical capsaicin in the treatment of pruritus. Int J Dermatol 2010;49(8):858–65.

174. Weisshaar E, Heyer G, Forster C, et al. Effect of topical capsaicin on the cutaneous reactions and itching to histamine in atopic eczema compared to healthy skin. Arch Dermatol Res 1998;290(6): 306–11.

175. Frolich M, Enk A, Diepgen TL, et al. Successful treatment of therapy-resistant pruritus in lichen amyloidosis with menthol. Acta Derm Venereol 2009;89(5):524–6.

176. Selescu T, Ciobanu AC, Dobre C, et al. Camphor activates and sensitizes transient receptor potential melastatin 8 (TRPM8) to cooling and icilin. Chem Senses 2013;38(7):563–75.

177. Sherkheli MA, Benecke H, Doerner JF, et al. Monoterpenoids induce agonist-specific desensitization of transient receptor potential vanilloid-3 (TRPV3) ion channels. J Pharm Pharm Sci 2009;12(1):116–28.

178. Valdes-Rodriguez R, Kaushik SB, Yosipovitch G. Transient receptor potential channels and dermatological disorders. Curr Top Med Chem 2013;13(3): 335–43.

179. Takashima Y, Daniels RL, Knowlton W, et al. Diversity in the neural circuitry of cold sensing revealed

by genetic axonal labeling of transient receptor potential melastatin 8 neurons. J Neurosci 2007; 27(51):14147–57.

180. Bromm B, Scharein E, Darsow U, et al. Effects of menthol and cold on histamine-induced itch and skin reactions in man. Neurosci Lett 1995;187(3): 157–60.

181. Peier AM, Moqrich A, Hergarden AC, et al. A TRP channel that senses cold stimuli and menthol. Cell 2002;108(5):705–15.

182. Galeotti N, Di Cesare Mannelli L, Mazzanti G, et al. Menthol: a natural analgesic compound. Neurosci Lett 2002;322(3):145–8.

183. Haught JM, Jukic DM, English JC 3rd. Hydroxyethyl starch-induced pruritus relieved by a combination of menthol and camphor. J Am Acad Dermatol 2008;59(1):151–3.

184. Panahi Y, Davoodi SM, Khalili H, et al. Phenol and menthol in the treatment of chronic skin lesions following mustard gas exposure. Singapore Med J 2007;48(5):392–5.

185. Yosipovitch G, Szolar C, Hui XY, et al. Effect of topically applied menthol on thermal, pain and itch sensations and biophysical properties of the skin. Arch Dermatol Res 1996;288(5–6):245–8.

186. Wilkinson SM, Beck MH. Allergic contact dermatitis from menthol in peppermint. Contact Dermatitis 1994;30(1):42–3.

187. Patel T, Yosipovitch G. Therapy of pruritus. Expert Opin Pharmacother 2010;11(10):1673–82.

188. Hatem S, Attal N, Willer JC, et al. Psychophysical study of the effects of topical application of menthol in healthy volunteers. Pain 2006;122(1–2):190–6.

189. Yosipovitch G, Maibach HI, Rowbotham MC. Effect of EMLA pre-treatment on capsaicin-induced burning and hyperalgesia. Acta Derm Venereol 1999;79(2):118–21.

190. Shuttleworth D, Hill S, Marks R, et al. Relief of experimentally induced pruritus with a novel eutectic mixture of local anaesthetic agents. Br J Dermatol 1988;119(4):535–40.

191. Sandroni P. Central neuropathic itch: a new treatment option? Neurology 2002;59(5):778–9.

192. Layton AM, Cotterill JA. Notalgia paraesthetica–report of three cases and their treatment. Clin Exp Dermatol 1991;16(3):197–8.

193. Allenby CF, Johnstone RS, Chatfield S, et al. PERINAL–a new no-touch spray to relieve the symptoms of pruritus ani. Int J Colorectal Dis 1993;8(4):184–7.

194. Kopecky EA, Jacobson S, Bch MB, et al. Safety and pharmacokinetics of EMLA in the treatment of postburn pruritus in pediatric patients: a pilot study. J Burn Care Rehabil 2001;22(3):235–42.

195. Gaudy-Marqueste C, Jouhet C, Castelain M, et al. Contact allergies in haemodialysis patients: a prospective study of 75 patients. Allergy 2009;64(2): 222–8.

196. O'Sullivan SE, Kendall DA. Cannabinoid activation of peroxisome proliferator-activated receptors: potential for modulation of inflammatory disease. Immunobiology 2010;215(8):611–6.

197. Godlewski G, Offertaler L, Wagner JA, et al. Receptors for acylethanolamides-GPR55 and GPR119. Prostaglandins Other Lipid Mediat 2009; 89(3–4):105–11.

198. Aloe L, Leon A, Levi-Montalcini R. A proposed autacoid mechanism controlling mastocyte behaviour. Agents Actions 1993;39 Spec No:C145–7.

199. Slutsky JB, Clark RA, Remedios AA, et al. An evidence-based review of the efficacy of coal tar preparations in the treatment of psoriasis and atopic dermatitis. J Drugs Dermatol 2010;9(10):1258–64.

200. van der Valk PG, Snater E, Verbeek-Gijsbers W, et al. Out-patient treatment of atopic dermatitis with crude coal tar. Dermatology 1996;193(1):41–4.

201. Munkvad M. A comparative trial of Clinitar versus hydrocortisone cream in the treatment of atopic eczema. Br J Dermatol 1989;121(6):763–6.

202. Backonja M, Glanzman RL. Gabapentin dosing for neuropathic pain: evidence from randomized, placebo-controlled clinical trials. Clin Ther 2003; 25(1):81–104.

203. Scheinfeld N. The role of gabapentin in treating diseases with cutaneous manifestations and pain. Int J Dermatol 2003;42(6):491–5.

204. Matsuda KM, Sharma D, Schonfeld AR, et al. Gabapentin and pregabalin for the treatment of chronic pruritus. J Am Acad Dermatol 2016;75(3): 619–25.e6.

205. Yang RH, Wang WT, Chen JY, et al. Gabapentin selectively reduces persistent sodium current in injured type-A dorsal root ganglion neurons. Pain 2009;143(1–2):48–55.

206. Li Z, Taylor CP, Weber M, et al. Pregabalin is a potent and selective ligand for $\alpha(2)\delta$-1 and $\alpha(2)\delta$-2 calcium channel subunits. Eur J Pharmacol 2011;667(1–3):80–90.

207. Quintero JE, Dooley DJ, Pomerleau F, et al. Amperometric measurement of glutamate release modulation by gabapentin and pregabalin in rat neocortical slices: role of voltage-sensitive Ca2+ $\alpha2\delta$-1 subunit. J Pharmacol Exp Ther 2011; 338(1):240–5.

208. Fehrenbacher JC, Taylor CP, Vasko MR. Pregabalin and gabapentin reduce release of substance P and CGRP from rat spinal tissues only after inflammation or activation of protein kinase C. Pain 2003; 105(1–2):133–41.

209. Bueller HA, Bernhard JD, Dubroff LM. Gabapentin treatment for brachioradial pruritus. J Eur Acad Dermatol Venereol 1999;13(3):227–8.

210. Jagdeo J, Kroshinsky D. A case of post-herpetic itch resolved with gabapentin. J Drugs Dermatol 2011;10(1):85–8.

211. Gunal AI, Ozalp G, Yoldas TK, et al. Gabapentin therapy for pruritus in haemodialysis patients: a randomized, placebo-controlled, double-blind trial. Nephrol Dial Transplant 2004;19(12):3137–9.

212. Yue J, Jiao S, Xiao Y, et al. Comparison of pregabalin with ondansetron in treatment of uraemic pruritus in dialysis patients: a prospective, randomized, double-blind study. Int Urol Nephrol 2015;47(1):161–7.

213. Aune TM, McGrath KM, Sarr T, et al. Expression of 5HT1a receptors on activated human T cells. Regulation of cyclic AMP levels and T cell proliferation by 5-hydroxytryptamine. J Immunol 1993;151(3): 1175–83.

214. Meredith EJ, Chamba A, Holder MJ, et al. Close encounters of the monoamine kind: immune cells betray their nervous disposition. Immunology 2005;115(3):289–95.

215. Slominski A, Pisarchik A, Zbytek B, et al. Functional activity of serotoninergic and melatoninergic systems expressed in the skin. J Cell Physiol 2003; 196(1):144–53.

216. Morita T, McClain SP, Batia LM, et al. HTR7 mediates serotonergic acute and chronic itch. Neuron 2015;87(1):124–38.

217. Stimmel GL, Dopheide JA, Stahl SM. Mirtazapine: an antidepressant with noradrenergic and specific serotonergic effects. Pharmacotherapy 1997;17(1):10–21.

218. Cevikbas F, Steinhoff M, Ikoma A. Role of spinal neurotransmitter receptors in itch: new insights into therapies and drug development. CNS Neurosci Ther 2011;17(6):742–9.

219. Stander S, Siepmann D, Herrgott I, et al. Targeting the neurokinin receptor 1 with aprepitant: a novel antipruritic strategy. PLoS One 2010;5(6):e10968.

220. Booken N, Heck M, Nicolay JP, et al. Oral aprepitant in the therapy of refractory pruritus in erythrodermic cutaneous T-cell lymphoma. Br J Dermatol 2011;164(3):665–7.

221. Stander S, Schmelz M. Chronic itch and pain–similarities and differences. Eur J Pain 2006;10(5):473–8.

222. Hagermark O. Peripheral and central mediators of itch. Skin Pharmacol 1992;5(1):1–8.

223. Ko MC, Naughton NN. An experimental itch model in monkeys: characterization of intrathecal morphine-induced scratching and antinociception. Anesthesiology 2000;92(3):795–805.

224. Monroe EW. Efficacy and safety of nalmefene in patients with severe pruritus caused by chronic urticaria and atopic dermatitis. J Am Acad Dermatol 1989;21(1):135–6.

225. Sullivan JR, Watson A. Naltrexone: a case report of pruritus from an antipruritic. Australas J Dermatol 1997;38(4):196–8.

226. Dawn AG, Yosipovitch G. Butorphanol for treatment of intractable pruritus. J Am Acad Dermatol 2006; 54(3):527–31.

227. Umeuchi H, Togashi Y, Honda T, et al. Involvement of central mu-opioid system in the scratching behavior in mice, and the suppression of it by the activation of kappa-opioid system. Eur J Pharmacol 2003;477(1):29–35.

228. Kardon AP, Polgár E, Hachisuka J, et al. Dynorphin acts as a neuromodulator to inhibit itch in the dorsal horn of the spinal cord. Neuron 2014;82(3): 573–86.

229. Mettang T. Uremic Itch Management. Curr Probl Dermatol 2016;50:133–41.

230. Yosipovitch G, Greaves MW, Schmelz M. Itch. Lancet 2003;361(9358):690–4.

231. Papoiu AD, Kraft RA, Coghill RC, et al. Butorphanol suppression of histamine itch is mediated by nucleus accumbens and septal nuclei: a pharmacological fMRI study. J Invest Dermatol 2015;135(2): 560–8.

232. Vieira BL, Lim NR, Lohman ME, et al. Complementary and alternative medicine for atopic dermatitis: an evidence-based review. Am J Clin Dermatol 2016;17(6):557–81.

233. Nilsson HJ, Levinsson A, Schouenborg J. Cutaneous field stimulation (CFS): a new powerful method to combat itch. Pain 1997;71(1):49–55.

234. Pfab F, Hammes M, Backer M, et al. Preventive effect of acupuncture on histamine-induced itch: a blinded, randomized, placebo-controlled, crossover trial. J Allergy Clin Immunol 2005;116(6): 1386–8.

235. Belgrade MJ, Solomon LM, Lichter EA. Effect of acupuncture on experimentally induced itch. Acta Derm Venereol 1984;64(2):129–33.

236. Lundeberg T, Bondesson L, Thomas M. Effect of acupuncture on experimentally induced itch. Br J Dermatol 1987;117(6):771–7.

237. Pfab F, Huss-Marp J, Gatti A, et al. Influence of acupuncture on type I hypersensitivity itch and the wheal and flare response in adults with atopic eczema - a blinded, randomized, placebo-controlled, crossover trial. Allergy 2010;65(7): 903–10.

238. Pfab F, Kirchner MT, Huss-Marp J, et al. Acupuncture compared with oral antihistamine for type I hypersensitivity itch and skin response in adults with atopic dermatitis: a patient- and examiner-blinded, randomized, placebo-controlled, crossover trial. Allergy 2012;67(4):566–73.

239. Lee KC, Keyes A, Hensley JR, et al. Effectiveness of acupressure on pruritus and lichenification associated with atopic dermatitis: a pilot trial. Acupunct Med 2012;30(1):8–11.

240. Napadow V, Li A, Loggia ML, et al. The brain circuitry mediating antipruritic effects of acupuncture. Cereb Cortex 2014;24(4):873–82.

241. Chida Y, Steptoe A, Hirakawa N, et al. The effects of psychological intervention on atopic dermatitis.

A systematic review and meta-analysis. Int Arch Allergy Immunol 2007;144(1):1–9.

242. Noren P. Habit reversal: a turning point in the treatment of atopic dermatitis. Clin Exp Dermatol 1995; 20(1):2–5.

243. Lavda AC, Webb TL, Thompson AR. A meta-analysis of the effectiveness of psychological interventions for adults with skin conditions. Br J Dermatol 2012;167(5):970–9.

244. Ehlers A, Stangier U, Gieler U. Treatment of atopic dermatitis: a comparison of psychological and dermatological approaches to relapse prevention. J Consult Clin Psychol 1995;63(4):624–35.

245. Schachner L, Field T, Hernandez-Reif M, et al. Atopic dermatitis symptoms decreased in children following massage therapy. Pediatr Dermatol 1998; 15(5):390–5.

246. Saeedi M, Morteza-Semnani K, Ghoreishi MR. The treatment of atopic dermatitis with licorice gel. J Dermatolog Treat 2003;14(3):153–7.

247. Schempp CM, Windeck T, Hezel S, et al. Topical treatment of atopic dermatitis with St. John's wort cream–a randomized, placebo controlled, double blind half-side comparison. Phytomedicine 2003; 10(Suppl 4):31–7.

248. Sheehan MP, Rustin MH, Atherton DJ, et al. Efficacy of traditional Chinese herbal therapy in adult atopic dermatitis. Lancet 1992;340(8810):13–7.

249. Cheng HM, Chiang LC, Jan YM, et al. The efficacy and safety of a Chinese herbal product (Xiao-Feng-San) for the treatment of refractory atopic dermatitis: a randomized, double-blind, placebo-controlled trial. Int Arch Allergy Immunol 2011;155(2):141–8.

250. Fung AY, Look PC, Chong LY, et al. A controlled trial of traditional Chinese herbal medicine in Chinese patients with recalcitrant atopic dermatitis. Int J Dermatol 1999;38(5):387–92.

251. Evangelista MT, Abad-Casintahan F, Lopez-Villafuerte L. The effect of topical virgin coconut oil on SCORAD index, transepidermal water loss, and skin capacitance in mild to moderate pediatric atopic dermatitis: a randomized, double-blind, clinical trial. Int J Dermatol 2014;53(1):100–8.

252. Lee J, Bielory L. Complementary and alternative interventions in atopic dermatitis. Immunol Allergy Clin N Am 2010;30(3):411–24.

253. Anstey A, Quigley M, Wilkinson JD. Topical evening primrose oil as treatment for atopic eczema. J Dermatolog Treat 1990;(4):199–201.

254. Kanehara S, Ohtani T, Uede K, et al. Clinical effects of undershirts coated with borage oil on children with atopic dermatitis: a double-blind, placebo-controlled clinical trial. J Dermatol 2007;34(12):811–5.

255. Bamford JT, Ray S, Musekiwa A, et al. Oral evening primrose oil and borage oil for eczema. Cochrane Database Syst Rev 2013;(4):CD004416.

Atopic Dermatitis
Racial and Ethnic Differences

Adeline Mei-Yen Yong, MRCP (UK)[a], Yong-Kwang Tay, FRCP (Lond)[b],*

KEYWORDS

- Atopic dermatitis • Eczema • Ethnic • Patterns • Trends

KEY POINTS

- Atopic dermatitis (AD) affects approximately 20% of schoolchildren in developed countries and approximately 3% of adults worldwide.
- Adult-onset AD is not uncommon, with a prevalence of 11% to 13% in some countries, for example, Singapore, Malaysia, and Sweden.
- Although the prevalence of AD is increasing in developing countries, the prevalence has stabilized in the developed countries.
- Erythema is not as pronounced on darker skin and may appear violaceous, which presents an obstacle to a physician making a diagnosis or assessing the severity of disease.
- Follicular or papular eczema and postinflammatory dyspigmentation are common in patients of color.

The severity and prevalence of AD may be increased in certain racial/ethnic populations, especially among blacks/African Americans. Erythema may be difficult to assess in patients with more darkly pigmented skin. Follicular or papular eczema and postinflammatory dyspigmentation are common in patients of color. Variations in the epidemiology of AD between different countries and ethnic groups may be due to differences in genetic predisposition, environmental, and socioeconomic factors.

INTRODUCTION

AD (or eczema) is a common inflammatory skin condition characterized by recurrent episodes of pruritus and a chronic, relapsing course. Having a persistent itch-scratch cycle, AD is associated with numerous complications, including secondary infections as well as significant comorbidities.[1–3] There is an impactful global health care economic burden associated with AD, on which interesting ethnic/racial trends can be observed.[4]

AD affects up to 20% of children and 3% of adults worldwide.[5] Recent data show that the prevalence of AD is still increasing globally, especially in low-income countries. Phase One of the International Study of Asthma and Allergies in Childhood (ISAAC) demonstrated a significant difference in the prevalence and incidence of AD both within countries and between geographic areas.[6] Scandinavia, Northern and Western Europe, Australasia, and urban areas in Africa suffered from the highest prevalence rates, whereas those in Eastern Europe, the Middle East, China, and Central Asia showed the lowest rates of prevalence. The reasons for such striking worldwide geographic variability in the epidemiology of AD are still unclear. Along with

Disclosure Statement: The authors have nothing to disclose.
[a] Department of Dermatology, National University Health System, 5 Lower Kent Ridge Road, Singapore 119074, Singapore; [b] Department of Dermatology, Changi General Hospital, 2 Simei Street 3, Singapore 529889, Singapore
* Corresponding author.
E-mail address: Yong_kwang_tay@cgh.com.sg

0733-8635/17/© 2017 Elsevier Inc. All rights reserved.

underlying genetic disposition, these variations have been attributed in part to environmental factors, including urbanization, climate, diet, aeroallergens, and infections.[7]

Elucidating the racial disparity and epidemiology of AD will spur efforts to identify modifiable risk factors, which can contribute toward disease prevention. As such, the authors review advancements in AD epidemiology, including interracial and ethnic differences, reasons for such disparity, variability of clinical presentation, and disease severity.

DIAGNOSIS AND DEFINITION

Epidemiologic studies essentially rely on accurate definitions of a disease. AD demonstrates significant clinical variability and has proved a challenge for the establishment of accurate diagnostic criteria. The first set of standardized diagnostic criteria was developed by Hanifin and Rajka in 1980, in which affected patients must possess at least 3 major and 3 minor criteria to satisfy a diagnosis of AD[8] (**Box 1**). The United Kingdom Working Party revision of 1990 furthered the development of a standardized criteria, which revealed a sensitivity of 87.9% and a specificity of 92.8% when evaluated in a hospital outpatient setting[9] (**Box 2**). This was generally limited, however, to those with mild to moderate forms of typical AD. In clinical practice, diagnosis is often established based on a pruritic relapsing condition in typical locations, including the neck, face, and extensor surfaces in children and infants.

RACIAL DISPARITY

The ISAAC, an international multicountry cross-sectional survey of school children, was conducted to investigate the epidemiology, geographic variability, and trends in the prevalence of asthma, rhinitis, and AD.[10] The ISAAC Phase One study was conducted in the early to mid-1990s. The ISAAC Phase Three was carried out approximately 7 years later using the same methodology and survey questionnaire to monitor the evolution in the prevalence of these disorders. This follow-up study involved 193,404 children ages 6 years to 7 years from 66 centers in 37 countries and 304,679 children ages 13 years to 14 years from 106 centers in 56 countries. Odhiambo and colleagues[11] analyzed data from the study and found a wide variation in prevalence values worldwide, from 0.9% in India to 22.5% in Ecuador at ages 6 years to 7 years and from 0.2% in China to 24.6% in Colombia at

| **Box 1** |
| **Hanifin and Rajka's diagnostic criteria for atopic dermatitis** |

Major criteria (must have at least 3)

Pruritus

Typical morphology and distribution

Adults: flexural lichenification or linearity

Children and infants: involvement of facial and extensor

Surfaces

Chronic or relapsing dermatitis

Personal or family history of atopy

Minor criteria (must have at least 3)

Xerosis

Ichthyosis/keratosis pilaris/palmer hyperlinearity

Immediate (type 1) skin test reactivity

Elevated serum IgE

Early age at onset

Tendency to skin infections (*Staphylococcus aureus*, herpes simplex)/impaired cellular immunity

Hand/foot dermatitis

Nipple eczema

Conjunctivitis

Dennie-Morgan fold

Keratoconus

Anterior subcapsular cataracts

Orbital darkening

Facial pallor/erythema

Pityriasis alba

Anterior neck folds

Itch when sweating

Intolerance to wool and lipid solvents

Perifollicular accentuation

Food intolerance

Course influenced by environmental/emotional factors

White demographic/delayed blanch

From Hanifin JM, Rajka G. Diagnostic features of atopic dermatitis. Acta Derm Venereol (Stockh) 1980;92(Suppl):45; with permission.

ages 13 years to 14 years. This study, along with other smaller population-based and community-based studies, suggests an overall higher AD prevalence in wealthier, developed nations compared with poorer, developing nations.[12–15]

ETHNIC VARIATION IN THE EAST

In the Asia-Pacific region, the 12-month prevalence of AD in children ages 13 years to 14 years was reported to be as high as 9% in Malaysia and Singapore and as low as 0.9% in China.[11] China demonstrated the lowest AD prevalence in the world. The reasons for these differences in AD prevalence are poorly understood, but industrialization and socioeconomic factors have been implicated.[15–22] Significantly, ISAAC Phase Three also highlighted the Asia-Pacific as an area of increasing AD prevalence. Of the 44 centers with an increase in prevalence, 10 were from the Asia-Pacific, hence putting this region second to Western Europe for centers with an increase in AD prevalence.

In Singapore, data derived from the ISAAC surveys indicated a modest increase in prevalence of AD among the age groups studied but an increased severity of symptoms in the 12-year to 15-year age group.[23] This is further supported by a cross-sectional epidemiologic study by Tay and colleagues[24] involving 12,323 students In SIngapore (7-year, 12-year, and 16-year age groups), reporting a prevalence of AD of 20.8%, a frequency markedly higher than that reported in younger age groups.[25,26] A recent community-based study of 681 randomly selected residents dwelling in public housing in Singapore showed a prevalence of AD of 20.6% in children (MJA Koh, personal communication, 2016) suggesting that the prevalence of AD in developed countries like Singapore has stabilized and is no longer increasing.

AGE DISPARITY

The diagnosis of AD is established by 1 year in 60% to 65% and by 5 years of age in 85% to 90% of children who have the disease.[27,28] Subsequently, up to a third of children have eczema that persists into adulthood.[29] Infantile AD is characterized by erythematous, oozing, excoriated plaques on the cheeks (sparing the nose), scalp, trunk, and extensor surfaces. In contrast, adult AD often presents as eczema of the hands and feet.

The prevalence of adult AD in the Western population was assessed to range from 1% to 3%.[30,31] In contrast, the prevalence of adult AD among Asian populations seems higher.

Saeki and colleagues[32] evaluated the prevalence of AD in Japanese adults at Kinki University and Asahikawa Medical College. A total of 2137 adult patients were examined. The prevalence of AD was 6.1% overall, and 10.5%, 7.8%, 3.9%, and 2.5%, respectively, for those in their 20s, 30s, 40s, and 50s/60s.

Sugiura and colleagues[13] compared the disease prevalence of AD in Japan and found that in 1967, 73.9% of patients with AD were children ages 0 to 9 years at the Branch Hospital of the University of Tokyo, but this figure gradually dropped to 23.4% by 1996. On the contrary, the percentage of adult patients ages 20 to 29 years with AD was 3.1% in 1967 and markedly increased to 38.7% by 1996.

In the same vein, the pattern of AD in Singapore demonstrates a significant proportion of adult-onset AD, with 13.6% of the study cohort having a later onset of symptoms above 21 years of age.[33] Findings were similar to another study carried out in Malaysia, where 13% of the patients had onset of AD after the age of 21 years.[34] The recent community-based study of public housing residents in Singapore showed similar trends: a prevalence of AD of 11.1% in adults.

In contrast, a lower prevalence of AD among Korean adults was reported by Kim and colleagues[35]: 2.6% overall, and 2.4%, 4.5%, 3.2%, 1.2%, and 0.4%, respectively, for those in their 10s/20s, 30s, 40s, 50s, and 60s and older.

In analyzing the data presented by Ronmark and colleagues[36] involving 18,087 adults from Sweden, an incidence of AD of 11.5% (16–75 years) was found, which suggests that adult AD may not be uncommon worldwide.

DIFFERENCES IN PHENOTYPE

AD essentially presents the same across different racial and ethnics groups. There exist several key differentiating factors, however, which are more typical among patients of darker skin types, that must be considered.

First, erythema is less obvious in skin of color and may often appear violaceous. This can present a challenge to physicians making a diagnosis and assessing the severity of AD. Erythema is a feature that is included in several scoring tools, including Scoring Atopic Dermatitis and Eczema Area and Severity Index. This may lead to a delay in diagnosis and treatment and a more severe disease progression.[37,38]

Second, patients with skin of color may manifest with follicular, papular, or lichenoid eczema as their primary disease phenotype (Fig. 1). Facial and eyelid dermatitis are more common in female Asians, infants, and teenagers.[39]

Nnoruka and colleagues[40] performed a 2- year prospective study of 1019 Nigerian black AD

Box 2
United Kingdom Working Party diagnostic criteria for atopic dermatitis

All patients must have an itchy skin condition in the last 12 months and have 3 or more of the following:

- History of involvement of the skin creases, such as antecubital, popliteal, dorsal ankles, or neck
- A personal history of asthma or hay fever (or history in first-degree relative in those under the age of 4)
- A history of generally dry skin during the last year
- Visible flexural dermatitis (or dermatitis of checks or forehead and outer limbs in children less than the age of 4
- Onset under the age of 2 (not used if child is under the age of 4)

From Williams HC, Burney PGL, Hay RJ, et al. The UK Working Party's diagnostic criteria for atopic dermatitis. I. Derivation of a minimum set of discriminators for atopic dermatitis. Br J Dermatol 1994;31:395–96; with permission.

patients against a control group of healthy individuals with no skin conditions. They found that the most frequent condition was xerosis (present in 71% of patients), which was significantly more common in patients than in controls (71% vs 4.3%; P<.005). Other minor features more common in the AD group than in the controls included papular lichenoid lesions (54% vs 2.1%; P<.001), infraorbital folds (49.2% vs 1.3%; P<.0001), palmar hyperlinearity (51.8% vs 0.8%; P<.001), and ichthyosis (21.4% vs 0%; P<.000). Less frequent minor features included forehead lichenification (10.7%), fissured heels (5.2%), palmar erythema (8.5%), nail pitting (4.3), knuckle dermatitis (3.8%), and pitted keratolysis (1.7%).

In a recent 2012 review article searching all available literature from January 1970 through August 2011 highlighting the differences in AD between African Americans and whites, Vachiramon and colleagues[38] found that scattered papular lesions on the extensors and trunk with annular configuration was commonly observed in black patients with AD. It was also observed that African Americans have a higher tendency to present with prurigo nodularis and lichenification than other ethnic groups.

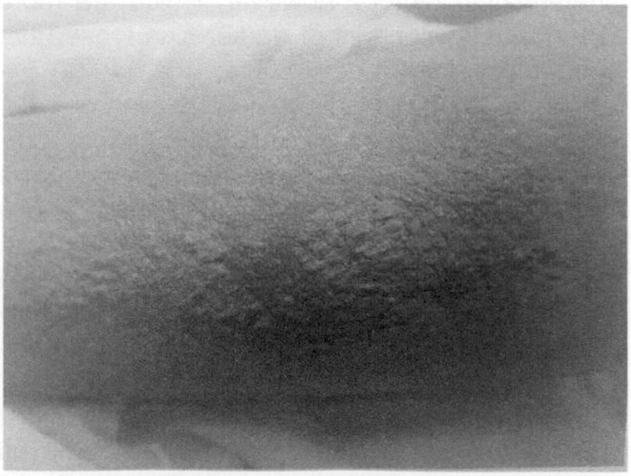

Persistent dyschromia or pigmentary alterations are almost always more pronounced in patients of darker skin when the lesions of AD resolve[38] (**Figs. 2** and **3**). Asian patients may present with sandpaper-like lesions on their extensor surfaces, wrist dermatitis, and hyperkeratotic papules as accompanying features.[41] African American children and adolescents often present with lesions on the extensor surfaces of the body as opposed to the usual traditional presentation of flexural involvement.[42] Dennie-Morgan lines are more commonly noted in patients of color, even in those without AD.[43]

DISTRIBUTION

The study of Nigerian patients with AD found that the extensors of the joints were most affected, with rash found in 70.3% of AD patients, whereas 51.8% had rash in the antecubital fossa and

Fig. 1. Lichenoid atopic dermatitis on the forearm of a Hispanic man. (*From* Berkowitz AC, Silverberg JI. Atopic dermatitis in pediatric skin of color. In: Silverberg NB, Durán-McKinster C, Tay YK, editors. Pediatric Skin of Color. New York: Springer; 2015. p. 270; with permission.)

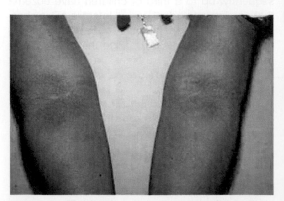

Fig. 2. Flexural eczema with prominent postinflammatory hyperpigmentation.

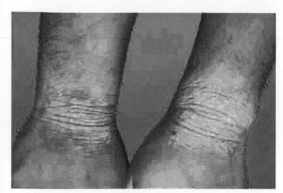

Fig. 3. Lichenified plaques of dermatitis with prominent postinflammatory hypopigmentation.

49.3% on the extensor surface of the elbow joints. The age group 0 to 3 years often showed a predominantly extensor pattern, whereas in the age group greater than 3 years to 18 years the flexural pattern was more common.

In addition, patients with perioral distribution were mainly children, whereas the older patients exhibited eczema on their hands and feet.

OTHER FEATURES

In a previous 2008 study, lesions that are nearly indistinguishable from classic lichen planus (lichen planus–like AD) were found more common in African Americans with AD.[44] Compared with classic lichen planus, in these patients the distribution of lichen planus–like AD was predominantly on the extensors and there was limited mucosal or genital involvement. The histopathology of such lesions revealed spongiosis, mild superficial perivascular lymphocytic infiltration with occasional eosinophils, and scattered melanophages.

In addition, it can be difficult to discriminate erythema within the context of pigmented skin. A 2002 study examined the effect of inclusion versus exclusion of erythema scores on disease severity in black and white children with AD; the data, including erythema scores, showed a nonsignificantly lower risk of severe disease in black children, whereas a highly significantly greater risk of severe disease was found after exclusion of erythema score.[37] When evaluating dark-skinned patients, practitioners may need to rely on patients' reports of reddened skin, which may be a more reliable indication of erythema. Skin lesions of AD may result in persistent dyschromia or pigmentary alterations, which are almost always more pronounced in patients of racial and ethnic groups with darker skin.

DISEASE SEVERITY

In terms of disease severity, studies have found that African Americans/blacks and Hispanics tend to have greater AD severity compared with whites[37,38] (**Fig. 4**). Ben-Gashir and Hay from the United Kingdom showed that black children with AD are approximately 6 times more at risk of having severe AD than white children.[37] In that study, 50% of the black children's parents were unemployed, which was a much higher unemployment rate than in parents of white children. Poorer access to medical care may be another explanation for the high prevalence of severe disease in African American patients with AD. In addition, difficulties of assessment of erythema can lead to a delay in diagnosis and treatment, which results in greater disease severity at presentation.

SOCIOECONOMIC FACTORS

Higher socioeconomic class seems to correlate with increasing prevalence of AD among different races. Increased rates of AD have been reported with rising social class in Britain and Switzerland.[45] In the British study, the point-prevalence of AD at age 7 in the highest socioeconomic class was twice that in the lowest socioeconomic class. An increase in prevalence was also seen in those families who owned their residences compared with children whose families rented. Reasons for this disparity may be attributable to increased exposure to medical care, increased immunizations, a more allergenic home environment, and smaller family size.[46,47]

GENETIC FACTORS

The role of genetics as an important risk factor for AD was first identified in observation studies, describing a positive parental history in AD patients, and in twin studies, showing a higher

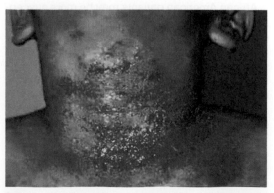

Fig. 4. Infected AD with oozing, erosions, and crusting.

concordance rate in monozygotic twins compared with dizygotic twins.[48]

The recent discovery of filaggrin gene (FLG) mutations associated with AD lends support for the role of genetic predisposition for AD. Filaggrin has a crucial role in skin barrier integrity. It is an important epidermal protein that is needed for the formation of the corneocytes as well as the generation of intracellular metabolites, which contribute to stratum corneum hydration and pH of the skin; 10% of the Western population and 50% of AD patients carry mutations in the FLG gene, and 20 mutations in the FLG gene have been described so far.[49]

Other skin-related genes, such as SPINK5/ LEKT1, have also been identified as associated with AD, which further supports differences in genetic differences with racial variability.[50,51]

Genetic susceptibility among races is a possible explanation because studies have shown that filaggrin mutations have significantly lower prevalence in black populations.[49,52,53] Some investigators also hypothesized that there is greater transepidermal water loss, higher immunoglobulin E (IgE) serum levels, and larger mast cell granules in African Americans. It is likely that a constellation of genes involved in the immune system and skin barrier function interact to product the phenotypic racial differences seen in AD.

TREATMENT

The cornerstones of treatment of AD include protecting the integrity of the epidermal barrier via emollients, avoidance of trigger factors, and implementing gentle skin care. Topical anti-inflammatory agents, including corticosteroids and calcineurin inhibitors, are first-line options for AD, depending on the site and severity of involvement. Among patients of different ethnic groups, these principles apply. A few key considerations should, however, be kept in mind.

African American patients may be more susceptible to severe disease. Hence, they may require maintenance therapy and alternative therapies to gain control of their disease and keep it in remission.[54,55] In view of erythema as a less reliable factor for determining the severity of disease, it is important for physicians to be cognizant of this and appropriately assess the degree of disease severity for appropriate treatment to be given.

A study evaluating treatment practices of Southeast Asian dermatologists showed variable levels of familiarity with diagnostic criteria. Appropriate use of moisturizers, topical corticosteroids, antibiotics, and other therapies was less than ideal.[56] A clear knowledge of the diagnostic criteria, consistent use of moisturisers, and appropriate use of corticosteroids and systemic agents should be stressed in these populations.

SUMMARY

The profile and pattern of AD is a complex and fascinating topic with wide variations in the prevalence between different countries. These differences may be due to an interplay of genetic predisposition; environmental factors, such as urbanization; and socioeconomic factors. Additionally, AD in darker patients tend to be follicular or papular, of increased severity, and with prominent postinflammatory dyspigmentation.

REFERENCES

1. Silverberg JI, Simpson EL. Association between severe eczema in children and multiple comorbid conditions and increased healthcare utilization. Pediatr Allergy Immunol 2013;24:476–86.
2. Silverberg JI, Silverberg NB. Childhood atopic dermatitis and warts are associated with increased risk of infection: a US population-based study. J Allergy Clin Immunol 2014;133:1041–7.
3. Simpson EL. Comorbidity in atopic dermatitis. Curr Dermatol Rep 2012;1:29–38.
4. Mancini AJ, Kaulback K, Chamlin SL. The socioeconomic impact of atopic dermatitis in the United States: a systematic review. Pediatr Dermatol 2008;25:1–6.
5. Nutten S. Atopic dermatitis: global epidemiology and risk factors. Ann Nutr Metab 2015;66(Suppl 1): 8–16.
6. Worldwide variation in prevalence of symptoms of asthma, allergic rhinoconjunctivitis, and atopic eczema: ISAAC. The International Study of Asthma and Allergies in Childhood (ISAAC) Steering Committee. Lancet 1998;351:1225–32.
7. Lee BW, Detzel PR. Treatment of childhood atopic dermatitis and economic burden of illness in Asia Pacific countries. Ann Nutr Metab 2015;66(Suppl 1):18–24.
8. Hanifin JM, Rajka G. Diagnostic features of atopic dermatitis. Acta Derm Venereol Suppl (Stockh) 1980;92:44–7.
9. Williams HC, Burney PG, Hay RJ, et al. The U.K. working party's diagnostic criteria for atopic dermatitis. I. Derivation of a minimum set of discriminators for atopic dermatitis. Br J Dermatol 1994;131: 383–96.
10. Asher MI, Keil U, Anderson HR, et al. International Study of Asthma and Allergies in Childhood (ISAAC): rationale and methods. Eur Respir J 1995;8:483–91.

11. Odhiambo JA, Williams HC, Clayton TO, et al. Global variations in prevalence of eczema symptoms in children from ISAAC phase three. J Allergy Clin Immunol 2009;124:1251–8.e23.

12. Xu F, Yan S, Li F, et al. Prevalence of childhood atopic dermatitis: an urban and rural community-based study in Shanghai, China. PLoS One 2012;7:e36174.

13. Sugiura H, Umemoto N, Deguchi H, et al. Prevalence of childhood and adolescent atopic dermatitis in a Japanese population: comparison with the disease frequency examined 20 years ago. Acta Derm Venereol 1998;78:293–4.

14. Kanwar AJ, De D. Epidemiology and clinical features of atopic dermatitis in India. Indian J Dermatol 2011;56:471–5.

15. Shaw TE, Currie GP, Koudelka CW, et al. Eczema prevalence in the United States: data from the 2003 National Survey of Children's Health. J Invest Dermatol 2011;131:67–73.

16. Bleiker TO, Shahidullah H, Dutton E, et al. The prevalence and incidence of atopic dermatitis in a birth cohort: the importance of a family history of atopy. Arch Dermatol 2000;136:274.

17. Strachan DP. Family size, infection and atopy: the first decade of the "hygiene hypothesis". Thorax 2000;55(Suppl 1):S2–10.

18. Tariq SM, Matthews SM, Hakim EA, et al. The prevalence of and risk factors for atopy in early childhood: a whole population birth cohort study. J Allergy Clin Immunol 1998;101:587–93.

19. Cogswell JJ, Mitchell EB, Alexander J. Parental smoking, breast feeding, and respiratory infection in development of allergic diseases. Arch Dis Child 1987;62:338–44.

20. Matsuoka S, Nakagawa R, Nakayama H, et al. Prevalence of specific allergic diseases in school children as related to parental atopy. Pediatr Int 1999;41:46–51.

21. Nicolaou N, Siddique N, Custovic A. Allergic disease in urban and rural populations: increasing prevalence with increasing urbanization. Allergy 2005;60:1357–60.

22. Weber AS, Haidinger G. The prevalence of atopic dermatitis in children is influenced by their parents' education: results of two cross-sectional studies conducted in Upper Austria. Pediatr Allergy Immunol 2010;21:1028–35.

23. Wang XS, Tan TN, Shek LP, et al. The prevalence of asthma and allergies in Singapore; data from two ISAAC surveys seven years apart. Arch Dis Child 2004;89:423–6.

24. Tay YK, Kong KH, Khoo L, et al. The prevalence and descriptive epidemiology of atopic dermatitis in Singapore school children. Br J Dermatol 2002; 146:101–6.

25. Tan TN, Lim DL, Lee BW, et al. Prevalence of allergy-related symptoms in Singaporean children in the second year of life. Pediatr Allergy Immunol 2005; 16:151–6.

26. Tan TN, Shek LP, Goh DY, et al. Prevalence of asthma and comorbid allergy symptoms in Singaporean preschoolers. Asian Pac J Allergy Immunol 2006;24:175–82.

27. Kay J, Gawkrodger DJ, Mortimer MJ, et al. The prevalence of childhood atopic eczema in a general population. J Am Acad Dermatol 1994;30:35–9.

28. Perkin MR, Strachan DP, Williams HC, et al. Natural history of atopic dermatitis and its relationship to serum total immunoglobulin E in a population-based birth cohort study. Pediatr Allergy Immunol 2004;15:221–9.

29. Ellis CN, Mancini AJ, Paller AS, et al. Understanding and managing atopic dermatitis in adult patients. Semin Cutan Med Surg 2012;31:S18–22.

30. de Bruin Weller MS, Rockmann H, Knulst AC, et al. Evaluation of the adult patient with atopic dermatitis. Clin Exp Allergy 2013;43:279–91.

31. Schmitt J, Bauer A, Meurer M. Atopic exzema in adulthood. Hautarzt 2008;59:841–50 [In German]; [quiz: 51].

32. Saeki H, Tsunemi Y, Fujita H, et al. Prevalence of atopic dermatitis determined by clinical examination in Japanese adults. J Dermatol 2006;33:817–9.

33. Tay YK, Khoo BP, Goh CL. The epidemiology of atopic dermatitis at a tertiary referral skin center in Singapore. Asian Pac J Allergy Immunol 1999;17: 137–41.

34. Jaafar RB, Pettit JH. Atopic eczema in a multiracial country (Malaysia). Clin Exp Dermatol 1993;18: 496–9.

35. Kim MJ, Kang TW, Cho EA, et al. Prevalence of atopic dermatitis among Korean adults visiting health service center of the Catholic Medical Center in Seoul Metropolitan Area, Korea. J Korean Med Sci 2010;25:1828–30.

36. Ronmark EP, Ekerljung L, Lotvall J, et al. Eczema among adults: prevalence, risk factors and relation to airway diseases. Results from a large-scale population survey in Sweden. Br J Dermatol 2012;166: 1301–8.

37. Ben-Gashir MA, Hay RJ. Reliance on erythema scores may mask severe atopic dermatitis in black children compared with their white counterparts. Br J Dermatol 2002;147:920–5.

38. Vachiramon V, Tey HL, Thompson AE, et al. Atopic dermatitis in African American children: addressing unmet needs of a common disease. Pediatr Dermatol 2012;29:395–402.

39. Kiken DA, Silverberg NB. Atopic dermatitis in children, part 1: epidemiology, clinical features, and complications. Cutis 2006;78:241–7.

40. Nnoruka EN. Current epidemiology of atopic dermatitis in south-eastern Nigeria. Int J Dermatol 2004;43: 739–44.

41. Lee HJ, Cho SH, Ha SJ, et al. Minor cutaneous features of atopic dermatitis in South Korea. Int J Dermatol 2000;39:337–42.

42. Williams HC, Pembroke AC, Forsdyke H, et al. London-born black Caribbean children are at increased risk of atopic dermatitis. J Am Acad Dermatol 1995; 32:212–7.

43. Rudzki E, Samochocki Z, Rebandel P, et al. Frequency and significance of the major and minor features of Hanifin and Rajka among patients with atopic dermatitis. Dermatology 1994;189:41–6.

44. Summey BT, Bowen SE, Allen HB. Lichen planus-like atopic dermatitis: expanding the differential diagnosis of spongiotic dermatitis. J Cutan Pathol 2008;35:311–4.

45. Williams HC, Strachan DP, Hay RJ. Childhood eczema: disease of the advantaged? BMJ 1994; 308:1132–5.

46. Gibbs S, Surridge H, Adamson R, et al. Atopic dermatitis and the hygiene hypothesis: a case-control study. Int J Epidemiol 2004;33:199–207.

47. Mercer MJ, Joubert G, Ehrlich RI, et al. Socioeconomic status and prevalence of allergic rhinitis and atopic eczema symptoms in young adolescents. Pediatr Allergy Immunol 2004;15:234–41.

48. Schultz Larsen FV, Holm NV. Atopic dermatitis in a population based twin series. Concordance rates and heritability estimation. Acta Derm Venereol Suppl (Stockh) 1985;114:159.

49. Palmer CN, Irvine AD, Terron-Kwiatkowski A, et al. Common loss-of-function variants of the epidermal barrier protein filaggrin are a major predisposing factor for atopic dermatitis. Nat Genet 2006;38:441–6.

50. Barnes KC. An update on the genetics of atopic dermatitis: scratching the surface in 2009. J Allergy Clin Immunol 2010;125:16–29 e1-11 [quiz: 30–1].

51. Moffatt MF. SPINK5: a gene for atopic dermatitis and asthma. Clin Exp Allergy 2004;34:325–7.

52. Margolis DJ, Apter AJ, Gupta J, et al. The persistence of atopic dermatitis and filaggrin (FLG) mutations in a US longitudinal cohort. J Allergy Clin Immunol 2012;130:912–7.

53. Garrett JP, Hoffstad O, Apter AJ, et al. Racial comparison of filaggrin null mutations in asthmatic patients with atopic dermatitis in a US population. J Allergy Clin Immunol 2013;132:1232–4.

54. Grim K, Rosen T. Inflammatory disorders with unique clinical features. In: Alexis AF, Barbosa VH, editors. Skin of color: a practical guide to dermatologic diagnosis and treatment. New York: Springer; 2013. p. 45–90.

55. Silverberg N. Dermatologic disorders in children of color. In: Alexis AF, Barbosa VH, editors. Skin of color: a practical guide to dermatologic diagnosis and treatment. New York: Springer; 2013. p. 327–50.

56. Chan YC, Tay YK, Sugito TL, et al. A study on the knowledge, attitudes and practices of Southeast Asian dermatologists in the management of atopic dermatitis. Ann Acad Med Singapore 2006;35: 794–803.

Index

Note: Page numbers of article titles are in **boldface** type.

Dermatol Clin 35 (2017) 403–408
http://dx.doi.org/10.1016/S0733-8635(17)30063-3
0733-8635/17

Printed and bound by CPI Group (UK) Ltd, Croydon, CR0 4YY

03/10/2024

01040384-0004